GOLD

AS A REMEDY IN DISEASE

GOLD

AS A REMEDY IN DISEASE:

NOTABLY IN SOME FORMS OF

ORGANIC HEART DISEASE,

Angina Pectoris, Melancholy, Tedium Vitæ,
Scrofula, Syphilis, Skin Disease,

AND AS AN

ANTIDOTE TO THE ILL EFFECTS OF MERCURY

By

JAMES COMPTON BURNETT, M.D., F.R.G.S.,

GYAN

Published by

Gyan Publishing House
5, Ansari Road
Daryaganj, New Delhi-110002
Phone: 011-47034999, 9811692060
E-mail: books@gyanbooks.com

Distribution Network
gyanbooks.com
India, USA, Canada, UK, Australia, France

ISBN : 978-81-212-6546-1 (PB)
First Published, 1879

2nd Impression 2022

Printed at: Gyan Press, Delhi.

GOLD
AS A REMEDY IN DISEASE
Author: JAMES COMPTON BURNETT

GOLD

AS A REMEDY IN DISEASE,

NOTABLY IN SOME FORMS OF

ORGANIC HEART DISEASE,

Angina Pectoris, Melancholy, Tedium Vitæ, Scrofula, Syphilis, Skin Disease,

AND AS AN

ANTIDOTE TO THE ILL EFFECTS OF MERCURY.

BY

JAMES COMPTON BURNETT, M.D., F.R.G.S.,

AUTHOR OF

"Natrum Muriaticum as Test of the Doctrine of Drug Dynamization."

" Aurum . . . Medicina Catholica in senibus et juvenibus."
—*Glauber*, 1651.

1879.

PREFACE.

IN reference to the subject of this little volume Hahnemann says, "*Das Gold hat grosse, unersetzliche Arznei-kraefte*") ("Gold has great remedial virtues, the place of which no other drug can supply"); and having myself used it in practice for several years, I have come to regard it in the same light: *I cannot do without it.* To my mind there are varieties of disease that *Gold*, and *Gold only*, will *cure*, and others that Gold, and Gold only, will alleviate *to the full extent of the possible;* and not a few of these varieties of disease are of the gravest nature. As a heart-remedy alone it claims the most earnest attention of every medical man.

In homœopathic practice it is neglected, and in allopathic practice it is practically unknown.

I claim for the following pages only that they constitute a rough Introduction to the Study of Gold as a Remedy in Disease.

J. C. B.

2, FINSBURY CIRCUS, LONDON, E.C.
February, 1879.

ERRATUM.

Page 54. *Instead of*—

Reading this, therefore, in connection with its other symptoms, I should class Aurum in *Grauvogl's Hydrogenoid Group.*

Read thus :—

Reading this, therefore, in connection with its other symptoms, we see why Grauvogl classed Aurum in his *Carbonitrogenoid Group.*

GOLD

AS A

REMEDY IN DISEASE.

FEW things affect mankind in more ways or more than the subject of this essay. But few of the drugs in our pharmacopœia possess such remarkable remedial properties; none are in general less known or less appreciated by both physician and patient than this metal in its physiological and therapeutical effects upon the human body.

This arises largely because—the metal being insoluble in its ordinary form—*it is taken for granted* that it *cannot* possess any remedial virtues.

But I shall hope to show in the course of these pages that Gold may be so subdivided that it becomes operative upon the living tissue of the body, and *thus acquires medicinal properties of the highest order*, and that, not merely in some functional disturbances of the organs and their parts, but also in states of deep-seated pathological changes that constitute complaints usually termed organic.

The various phases of thought in medicine have produced views of drugs and drug-action that differ widely from one another ; to some a drug simply cures because it is endowed with remedial virtues . . . *quia est in eo vertus dormitiva*, as Molière has it. Some consider that there are substances that are of a benign and kindly nature, and are present in creation only to be remedies for our diseases, which really amounts to the same thing; while other substances are in themselves hurtful to our bodies, simply, and altogether bad. In one word, there are good and evil substances considered in relation to our bodies; the good ones to heal, the bad ones to hurt.

But Nature is not thus childishly constituted; the same substance is either good, bad, or indifferent, according to how it is used, and according to the state of aggregation of its parts.

Two equivalents of hydrogen and one of oxygen, as water, will quench our thirst, act as a solvent to our food, with a few other constituents float about in our bodies as blood. Hail, ice, sleet, and snow are also only hydrogen and oxygen in the same proportion; they are practically only water, just the same as the steam that whirls us along in the train. We are not astonished at these things;

the most marvellous things cease to excite wonder after we have grown accustomed to them.

Tell the noble savage that snow, hail, ice, water, and steam are chemically the same, though physically and dynamically so different, and he will not fail to laugh at *your* ignorance! *He* knows better. Tell the mediocre medical mind that common table-salt* may be so subdivided by means of friction that it thereby becomes a most powerful and even dangerous† drug, and he will not fail to laugh at you! *He* knows better. Tell the same that Gold may be so subdivided by simple friction that it becomes an active remedy, second to none in its great power, and the same result follows; he laughs at you. *He* knows

* See "*Natrum Muriaticum* as Test of the Doctrine of Drug Dynamization" (London: E. Gould and Son, 1878), on this subject.

† Dangerous when administered to the *sick*.

better. 'Tis true he never tried, but *he* knows. But who should be angry at the poor savage for that he knoweth nought of? Civilisation will teach the untutored mind of the savage what difference of temperature and pressure may effect in the physical state of water—if he survive long enough.

The advance of general and medical knowledge will teach the untutored medical mind (*car il y a beaucoup de docteurs qui ne sont point doctes*), what trituration will do in the way of transforming a non-medicinal substance into a potent remedy, but it will, probably, not be the medical mind of the crude chirurgeons of the present day. *They* know better.

The subject we wish to introduce is, "*Gold: as a Remedy in Disease, notably in* (some forms of) *Organic Heart-Disease, Angina Pectoris, Melancholy,*

Tedium Vitæ, Scrofula, Syphilis, Skin Disease, and as an *Antidote to the Ill Effects of Mercury.*"

We will try to keep to our text.

It is now admitted on all sides that a true and thorough knowledge of a medicine can be obtained in only one way, viz., *by first testing it on the healthy.*

Why?

Because if you give a sick person, X, a dose of medicine of any kind, and there follow, say, six phenomena, how many and which of these were due to the drug, and how many and which were due to the disease? You cannot tell, and therefore you give it to a healthy person to find out.

Suppose we give thirty grains of powdered ipecacuanha root to a healthy person, we find it produces vomiting. That is a symptom of *Ipecacuanha;* all the symptoms produced by a drug on a healthy person constitute the pathogenesis, or proving, of that drug.

When we know all the physiological effects of a given drug, that is, its pathogenesis, we have a firm scientific basis to work upon. This pathogenetic material constitutes the means of curing disease by using it on the now well-known, but ill-comprehended, principle of similars.

But before coming to this point, it is, to say the least, very interesting to cast a glance back into the history of a drug to see what was thought of it by our fathers that have gone before us, and by our forefathers in the old times before them. By this means we learn the empirical uses of a drug, and can compare notes with those that have long since gone over to the majority, and thus we can satisfy ourselves whether they were right or wrong, and whether we know more than they knew on the subject, or whether indeed they knew many a useful thing that we have allowed to lapse into disuse or even oblivion. Therefore I shall treat my subject somewhat historically, and expect to show that all the medical wisdom we ween to possess on this subject did not originate with us of this generation.

If we have the history of the subject in a few outlines—just a silhouette—then the effects on the healthy, or pathogenesis, also only in outline, and then a few experiments on animals, we shall be able to fully appreciate that to which all this is only preliminary and introductory, viz., *Gold as a remedy in disease.*

To begin, then, with the first:—

The history of Gold begins very early in the records of our race; it is the first metal discovered by man, and also the first metal mentioned in the Bible.

The eleventh verse of the second chapter of Genesis reads: "The name of the first is Pison: that is it which compasseth the whole land of Havilah, where there is *Gold.*" Thus it is noticed even before Eve was created. This is, of course, some thousands of years ago. I need therefore not state that a complete history of Gold lies beyond the scope of this little work. The great Linné (Mat. Med.) writes its history in four words: *Vis politica, usus œconomicus.*

I propose going a little further than this.

Magpies, crows, and other thieving birds are attracted by its colour and its sheen, and hence a state of man in which Gold is unknown is hardly conceivable.

The first metallic instruments were made of Gold (Hoefer, Histoire de la Chimie).

In the 25th chapter of Exodus there is an account of dishes, spoons, bowls, etc., made of this metal, as every one knows.

The first trituration of Gold was made by Moses out of the remains of the golden calf of the Israelites, and he made the children of Israel drink it in water (Exodus, chap. xxxii. v. 20). Hence it is also the first *Aurum potabile* on record.

What the precise object of Moses was in thus dealing with the remains of the golden calf may be a fit matter for discussion; certainly a more efficient way of proving the nullity of a god could not be well devised. What the opinions of Biblical scholars on the subject may be I do not know. In medical works I have read the opinion that the golden calf was really made of wood, and only encased with Gold, and that causing the children of Israel to drink it was with the view of purifying them of their great sin of worshipping an idol.

Gold is constantly connected with the idea of purity and purification, as witness the expression, "Pure as gold."

At the risk of being irksome and of appearing pedantic, I shall give the sources of my information in many instances, and sometimes even give the original text when I think it best.

The first notice of Gold as a medicine known to me is that in Wiegleb's "History of Alchemy" (Historisch-Kritische Untersuchung der Alchemie, Weimar, 1777), p. 185, where he treats of the antiquity of chemistry amongst the Chinese, and according to which Gold was used by them medicinally 2500 B.C. I sometimes wonder how much *blague* is contained in these pretensions of the Chinese to such great antiquity.

All along the march of time, physicists have been seeking a *Perpetuum mobile*, mathematicians have been squaring the circle, and husbandmen trying to manure without dung; what wonder, then, that alchemists should have sought the philosopher's stone, and physicians a never-failing panacea!

Gold has more than once figured as the universal cure-all, as a veritable *elixir vitæ;* and it will indeed cure many diseases, as has been long known, and as I hope to show, but it has never been known to cure chryso-dypsia; at any rate I know of no such case on record.

It is wonderfully strange to read of the doings of the curious craft of alchemists, and nowhere more strange than in the works of that erratic genius and honest man Hohenheim, commonly called Paracelsus.

But, withal, the transmutation of

common metals into gold and silver, and the discovery of the true *lapis philosophorum*, run like a thread through them all. That such a gestation should have eventuated in the birth of chemistry is only another proof that good comes of all honest work. The alchemists called Gold the king of metals, *rex metallorum*, and the sun, *Sol.* We may fairly invert it, and say it is the metal of kings. The Greek αυρον is parent of the Latin *aurum*, and of the French *or;* the more usual Greek word is χρυσος. Dioscorides and Avicenna employed Gold as a remedy in the metallic state. Paracelsus used it with sublimate as a universal panacea, and called this *Calcinatio et solutio* "*solis.*"

For years I have tried to fix the date at which Gold was first used as an anti-syphilitic, but I must confess that I have been unable to do so.

It is pretty sure that Hahnemann thus used it, as it is so evidently homœopathic to some cases of this disease, but it did not originate with this great man.

Dr. Richard Hughes, in his remarkable work, "Pharmacodynamics," seems to ascribe it to Chrétien (meaning evidently Chrestien), but Chrestien certainly did not originate it. What Chrestien did would seem to be this: he first started a would-be new method of cure, "*Méthode par Absorption,*" very early in this century, and then this became, "*Méthode jatraleptice*" (*de l'an* xii.), and then (1811), "*De la méthode jatraleptique, etc., et sur un nouveau remède dans le traitement des maladies vénériennes et lymphatiques.*" He met with violent opposition from the profession, which had long abandoned the use of Gold in medicine (the ancient *Pulvis Auri, Tinctura Auri, Aurum potabile*, *Aurum potabile verum*, *Tinctura Solis*, *Tinctura aurea*, etc.), it having been so highly prized and praised by the alchemists, and long been the stock-in-trade of secret-mongers and quacks of all kinds, that it passed from being the *remède à la mode* into utter oblivion. This is the rock upon which lawless therapy has always stranded; at first a given drug is a "new remedy," then it is a wonderful medicine, and then a universal panacea, then it is not such a very good medicine after all, and finally it is accounted no good at all, is abandoned like an old mine, and venturous spirits set out in quest of another "new remedy," and so on in a veritable vicious circle.

Hahnemann gathered up the fragments, welded them together with the light of his law, and gave *fixity* to the whole. The *proof* of this lies in the fact that Gold has never ceased being used by the homœopaths, in cases judged appropriate, from his day to this, and that is some fifty years since. Be it therefore observed that I do not claim to resuscitate the dead when I call attention to this great polychrest. It is now essentially a homœopathic remedy, just as *Aconite* or *Belladonna,* not that the homœopaths originated its use (any more than that of *Aconite,* for instance), but they use it on a fixed principle, which reduces fits of fashion in the drug-treatment of disease to a minimum. M. Chrestien, as we have said, met with violent opposition, and this put him on his mettle ; and he set earnestly to work to explore this veritable therapeutic mine of Gold with the result that quite a school of men arose that one might fitly term "*Auralists,*" more especially amongst syphilidographers, and the movement culminated in the important work of M. Legrand, "*De l'Or, de son emploi dans le traitement de la syphilis récente et invétérée et dans celui des dartres syphilitiques; Du Mercure, de son inefficacité, et des dangers de l'administrer dans le traitement des mêmes maladies, etc.* Paris, 1828." Thus these auralists constituted one camp, and the old mercurialists the other; as if the one *excluded* the other! As if the fact of Gold being a good remedy in some forms of syphilis precluded *Mercury* from being equally good in some other forms of the same malady, or even in the same! Dr. X tells you pompously he does not believe in this or that remedy, but in the other; as if the purging of jalap prevented *Colocynth* from doing a similar thing!

But the auralist and anti-mercurialist, Legrand, did important pharmacological work, of which we shall make full use in these pages. M. Legrand's position is not the one I propose to defend in what follows; I purpose merely making use of his *facts*. Neither do I propose to join in the insane cry of the so-called anti-mercurialists; on the contrary, if I were reduced to one remedy in the treatment of the protean manifestations of this disease, I should certainly choose *Mercury*, for if there is any one thing certain in practical medicine, it is that *Mercury* is, *facile princeps*, the anti-syphilitic remedy. But the *dose?* Ay, *there's* the rub! To do the good without risking the harm is the true test.

Moreover, I do not propose to vaunt the use of Gold in this special disease, but rather to point out that it deserves a very much higher place in the *armamentarium* of the physician than is accorded to it in general. For centuries

Gold has been used with excellent effect in scrofula, heart-disease, skin diseases, dropsy, tedium vitæ, melancholia, and the Morbus Gallicus, or syphilis.

In the treatment of some heart diseases, some bone diseases, and of sarcocele, to know the medicinal value of Gold or to ignore it, is just the important difference between curing and failing. But, of course, the metal must be first triturated, so that it may become remedial.

In combination with *Mercury*, Gold has long been used as an anti-syphilitic, certainly as early as 1621, by J. Colle, and in 1623, as *Aurum vitæ*, by Planis Campi, in the pest, in *syphilis*, leprosy, dropsy, etc., as we read in the *Dictionnaire Universel de Matière Médicale*, of Mérat and De Lens.

And lying before me is old Glauber's "De Auri Tinctura, sive Auro Potabili Vero, etc.," Amsterdam, 1651, in which he distinctly recommends his tincture of Gold in the *Morbus Gallicus.* The same author also recommends it in leprosy, the pest, epilepsy, fevers, for promoting the menses, and in diseases of the uterus, and sterility. Further, he commends it very highly in dropsy, and concludes by apostrophising it as a *Medicina catholica in senibus et juvenibus.* And such it is.

Moreover, Mérat states that Pitcairn proposed, in 1714, powdered or leaf-gold as an anti-syphilitic in lieu of *Mercury.* This is about a century before M. Chrestien, of Montpellier. Again Timpe cites "Plencik: *Opera Medico-physica, Vindob,* 1762" and "Gmelin: *Apparatus Medicaminum, Goething,* 1795," on the same subject.

Finally, Mitchell, of New York, is quoted by Mérat before Chrestien. It is, however, only on the ground of priority that we must refuse honour to Chrestien's publications, as they undoubtedly mark a distinct era in the history of Gold as an anti-syphilitic, anti-venereal, and anti-scrofulosum. After the publication of Chrestien's works, the question, Is Gold a reliable anti-syphilitic? occupïed the medical mind of Europe for twenty years; to say that Gold has hardly been recognised, in this connection, outside of France, is incorrect. A mass of trustworthy evidence is collected by M. Legrand on the subject of the medicinal value of auric preparations. He gives a list of about eighty medical men of the time—auralists—who had tried Gold in syphilis and venereal diseases generally, and in scrofula and sarcocele, with a total number of 387 cases of these various diseases successfully treated by it, and comprising cases of recent origin, and treated with Gold only, as well as very inveterate ones that had resisted the action of *Mercury*, though other remedies were at times used with it. There is a later publication of M. Chrestien, Paris, 1821, entitled, "Recherches et observations sur les effets des preparations d'Or, du Docteur Chrestien, dans le traitement de plusieurs maladies ; et notamment dans celui des maladies syphilitiques. Par J. G. Niel, Docteur en Médecine de Montpellier, etc."

Niel was a Spanish practitioner of some position.

Lying before me is also, "De auri muriatica in morbis syphiliticis usu," which is an inaugural dissertation of L. B. Timpe, of Berlin (1834), and which I here only note, but shall hereafter have occasion to again refer to more fully.

The "*Dissertatio medica inauguralis de auro ejusque praeparatorum in medicina usu, auctore* J. D. Schepers, Groningae, 1838," shows conclusively that at the period of its date Gold was a thoroughly established remedy in Dutch hospitals, and was as such lectured upon by the teachers and highly commended in the same class of maladies.

In *De Methodis atque medicamenibus anti-syphiliticis* thesis of F. G. Sarfass, Berlin, 1816, p. 13, we read, "Nec auri usus deest in syphilidis therapia, Scotus Pitcairne (Girtanner, 3 Bd. p. 351. Diss. de ingressu morbi, qui venerea lues appellatur vulgo, in Pitcaïrnii dissertationibus. Amstelod, 1714), auro subtilissime alcoholisato in lue adhibito, melius et tutius quam hydrargyro hunce morbum sanari docet." But no mention is made of M. Chrestien. Clearly, then, the honour of first using Gold as an anti-syphilitic remedy cannot be claimed for M. Chrestien, although he vulgarised its use and originated the *Aurum muriaticum natronatum.* Perhaps I dwell more on this point than it deserves, but I am anxious to show that the assumption by certain writers of the honour of introducing this drug into the therapeutics of given ailments is wrongful. Nevertheless, I am unable to say positively *who first* used Gold in the treatment of syphilis; certain it is that Glauber recommends it in 1651, and in his *Tractatus de Medicina Universali sive Auro Potabili Vero* (a small tract in German and Latin mixed), Amsterdam, 1657, p. 69, he again asserts that it will cure the *Morbus Gallicus.*

Hence, to claim the introduction of *Aurum* into the therapeutics of syphilis for the homœopathic school, as do some, or for M. Chrestien, as do some modern writers, and as did many of M. Chrestien's immediate followers, is incorrect.

I have a strong feeling agàinst this system of robbing the dead of what is fairly due to their names.

The use of Gold in scrofula, in heart affections, in dyspnœa, and in mania is at least equally ancient with those other of its uses just indicated.

Strictly speaking, in Homœopathy no remedy is used as against any specific disease, but in any and every disease to the symptoms of which a given remedy is pathogenetically similar.

Still practical medicine, without a nosological nomenclature, is an *Unding*, and equally so practical pharmacology. All we have to bear in mind is that, *e.g.*, pneumonia is not an entity, but a generic term for a group of symptoms and a state of the organic tissues. I often wonder that such terms as *Morbus Auri*, *Morbus Aconiti*, *Morbus Chelidonii*, etc., are not more frequently met with in medical literature; they would be convenient, to say the least; they are used by Rademacherians, as followers of Paracelsus.

To say much more anent the medical history of *Aurum* might be tedious and unprofitable; but the historical part can hardly be avoided if we wish to be fair to the memories of the departed.

It is the great glory of Hahnemann to have introduced the systematic study of the effects of drugs in the healthy subject into medicine, thereby laying the very foundation of *any* system of Scientific Medicine. This is now admitted on all sides, except that every little chanticleer gets the credit of it rather than Hahnemann. The world is not yet capable of appreciating the herculean labours of this great teacher. The day will come when the *Hahnemannian Oration* will be the rendezvous of all that is great and good in the medical world. At present his lot is scorn, ridicule, slander, and contempt, and, worse than all, his life labour is daily filched from him by the pigmies of the hour.

But Nemesis lives, happily, through all time, and may tarry, but will surely overtake them. Awaiting this, it is for the small and persecuted body of the disciples of Hahnemann to follow in his wake, fearing neither ridicule, slander, nor hatred.

Our next step will be a consideration of the *Pathogenesis of Gold*, or an account of what Gold does when taken into the living body of the healthy. Here we are entirely upon homœopathic ground, for an account of the effects of metallic Gold upon the healthy human subject does not, I believe, exist in medical literature before the time of

Hahnemann, who first gives a proving* of *Aurum* in the fourth volume of his *Reine Arzeneimittellehre* (1825), and this is again given, with additions, in his *Chronische Krankheiten* (1835). Dr. Richard Hughes throws discredit upon these additional symptoms in these words: "The worth of these, according to the facts we have ascertained, is more than problematical" (Pharmacodynamics). What Dr. Hughes's facts are I do not know; the work of verifying Hahnemann seems to be undertaken by Dr. Hughes with a very light heart; now we require some one to verify Dr. Hughes. For that the latter may sometimes err also, is seen on the very same page, and indeed in the very same

* "Proving" is the English rendering of the German word *Pruefung*, meaning a trial, and is exclusively used in homœopathic literature, and is equivalent to *trial of a drug on a healthy organism*, *i.e.*, what it does.

paragraph, where he states that the symptoms of metallic Gold "were obtained from one- and two-hundred-grain doses of the first trituration" (see "Pharmacodynamics," 3rd edition, p. 153, § 2), which is incorrect.

If Dr. Hughes will kindly reach his *Chronische Krankheiten* from his library shelf and turn up the 217th page of the *Antipsorische Arzeneien* and glance at it again, he will, I think, agree with me that he has made an important mistake, inasmuch as the one and two hundred grains there mentioned were the quantities used in the entire provings of the individual provers, and not the "doses." Also that it was not precisely our "first trituration" that was used, as the proportion was 1 : 100 and not 1 : 99; this latter point is, of course, unimportant, but not so the former. It should also be stated that this one per cent. trituration was taken *dissolved in water.* Again, Dr. Hughes asserts that Gold does not affect the gums, which it certainly does.

I should not thus take upon myself to correct Dr. Hughes, for I owe my conviction of the truth of Homœopathy largely to a perusal of his beautifully written and most erudite works,* and I shall never be able to pay this great debt; but as he corrects his master, Hahnemann, I may perhaps be fairly forgiven for correcting mine. For my part I find Hahnemann so reliable and so exact that if my observations and his do not tally, I look again and am convinced of *my* error.

Dr. Taylor, F.R.S., of Guy's (on Poisons in Relation to Medical Jurisprudence and Medicine, 3rd edition, London, 1875, p. 493), says that nothing

* And to my friend, Dr. Hawkes, of Liverpool.

is known of the effects of Gold in the human subject.

Would this eminent man and learned author be very much surprised to learn that, just *Fifty Years* before the date of his book, one Samuel Hahnemann and *ten other medical men* carefully tried the effects of large doses of Gold upon *their own bodies* (not on rabbits and guinea-pigs, and dogs and cats, be it well understood, but on *themselves*)? How is it possible that such misstatements pass current? Because the spirit of Dr. Taylor's medical party *forbids the avowal* of any acquaintance with the writings of Hahnemann; the motto of this party is, "Nul n'aura de l'esprit que nous et nos amis."

But some have naughty notions of freethought in matters medical, and, to use an inelegant expression, chew their own cuds, and these *do* read Hahnemann;

some, having read the *Chronische Krankheiten* aforesaid, find it a most masterly production, full of sound learning, deep philosophical thought, true insight into Nature's ways in the maze of morbid phenomena that are the in-grip and the outcome of that hydra-headed monster *psora*, that in the times that be is just visible in the van of medical thought as the *Herpetic Diathesis.* We would respectfully commend a perusal of the *Chronische Krankheiten* to all medical men, of whatever shade of opinion. Allopath, homœopath, hydropath, eclectic—all should read it, and no man's medical education is so good but he may learn much by so doing.

For the purposes of this little book a simple sketch of the pathogenesis of *Aurum* in broad traits will be best. A bare list of all its symptoms is the province of an encyclopædia. In all it comprises 440 pathogenetic facts usually called symptoms—*i.e.*, symptoms of the drug-disease.

We say drug-disease in the sense of Paracelsus, who regarded drug-effect as an *infection*, being herein a forerunner of Hahnemann.

Triturated Leaf Gold, *Aurum foliatum*, was the substance used. Some of the experimenters—all healthy men—took as much as a hundred grains of a one per cent. trituration, and others as much as two hundred grains, dissolved in water. Whether they took the quantity in one single dose or in various doses is not distinctly stated, except as "*in der Prüfung*," and evidently this, with the context, means in divided parts.

Beginning with the sensorium, we note how some became *depressed in spirits*, *plaintive*, *tearful*, *melancholy*, *desirous of death*, *suicidal*, *restless*, *anxious*, and some *timid, irritable, disagreeable, getting into quite a rage at the least contradiction,* and *wanting to quarrel and going into violent passions.* In some the opposite state of *great hilarity* is noted: and in others *the two states alternate.*

One *sits moping in a corner,* desirous of being left alone, while another is *all vivacity,* and has a lively word for everybody.

In some *the memory* is rendered very *acute,* while in *others it becomes almost annihilated.*

Not only does Gold thus affect the brain, but it is a great disturber of the cranial circulation; there are *rushes of blood to the head and brain, headache, giddiness* and *hammering,* and *rustling noises in the head.*

And not only are the contents of the skull thus so materially disturbed in their states and functions, but the bony shell itself is profoundly affected in its life and being, as witness the *pains in the bones of the head, with tenderness on pressure,* and the *bony lumps* to be *felt under the hairy scalp.*

The *eyes,* too, are *powerfully* and *painfully* affected, and in one observer the *pupils* were at *first contracted* and *then dilated,* while the vision of another is interfered with; "*he sees indistinctly,*" and there is even *total loss of vision for a moment;* and finally Dr. Hermann is so affected that he *sees only with the lower half of his eyes, as if they were covered superiorly with something black* (see the eye cases later on), and then again he *cannot see anything distinctly, as everything seems double,* and thus objects get jumbled together.

There is a pustular *eruption on the face, neck, and chest,* the *parotid* and *submaxillary glands swell* and *are painful;* the *bones* of the *face* and *nose* are *tender* and *painful,* while the *wings of the nose* are *sore* and *inflamed*, and there is a *sore within them that scabs over.*

The *teeth pain* and are loose, the *gums are sore*, and *so is the throat;* there is an *offensive smell from the mouth* (one of the earliest uses of Gold was to correct foul *breath*), with *a good deal of saliva in the mouth* (the muriate produces inodorous (?) salivation).

The digestive tract is irritated and disturbed throughout; *uneasiness in the stomach*, amounting at times to a *sense of weight*, *pain*, or *swelling; stitches in the sides; nausea; retching; griping; colic; flatulence; flatulent colic; weight in the abdomen, with icy cold hands and feet; pressing in the right inguinal ring as if a hernia would protrude, an inguinal hernia protrudes with great pain; distention of the bowels with rumbling within; constipation, flatus, diarrhœa; stitches, burning and swelling of anal end of rectum;* in fact, the whole of the intestinal tube is irritated and fretted till it writhes and wriggles, protruding at the inguinal ring, and voiding its contents.

Nor are the kidneys exempt; there *is constant desire to micturate, the urine is like butter-milk,* and *more fluid is passed than is drunk* (its use in dropsy is very ancient).

The genital sphere is powerfully moved (in these experiments all adult males); a *long dormant appetite is roused* in one, and *generally great orgasm of the parts,* with *all* the known phenomena that *result therefrom.* Their various anatomical parts are fretted; stitches in the urethra and glans, with escape of prostatic secretion; the scrotum itches, the *right testis pains* as if bruised in one observer, and in *another observer* the *same* organ *becomes a tumid mass with pressive pain when touched or rubbed against from* 6 *to* 11 *p.m.*

Going back now to the respiratory

sphere, we note *all the symptoms of a running cold in the head*, and then *congestion and catarrh* of the *entire bronchial lining with the dry and humid stages* and *cough* with *dyspnœa* and *constriction of the thorax, or just the opposite*—viz., unusual freedom of breathing.

The symptoms of cardiac asthma are thus and in the following well depicted: *extreme tightness of the chest with difficult breathing at varying times, great weight on the chest, especially a heavy weight in the sternum.* This latter symptom points to *angina pectoris*, in which I have used it with marked success.

In view of its ancient reputation as a cordial,* the cardiac symptoms have a great interest. We read further: *In walking the heart seems to shake about as if it*

* "For gold in physic is a cordial,
Therefore he loved gold in special."
—*Chaucer.*

were loose; at times a single thump of the heart; palpitation of the heart; violent palpitation of the heart; a kind of restless anxiety, arising in the region of the heart, and driving him from one place to another, so that he cannot stay anywhere.

There are various *tearing stitch-like pains about the body*, and the *spine pained* one prover so much one morning that he *could not move hand or foot.*

There are *tearing pains in nearly all the joints*, and the *muscular system is considerably affected*, so also the *bones.*

There are *wheals in the skin of the lower extremities like nettle-rash that itch, are made worse by rubbing, and are worse out of doors.*

There is a *weary, tired pain in the head and in all the joints in the morning in bed that motion ameliorates.*

The arms and legs are numb and asleep in the morning on awaking. (I have cured this symptom, occurring in a middle-aged man, with Gold.)

There is *great liability to catch cold and great sensitiveness of the whole body to all kinds of pain, so that the very thought of pain is almost the pain itself.*

There is a good deal of *wakefulness by day* and *restlessness by night* with *bad dreams; "he often awakes in the night in a fright;" "he moans in his sleep."*

Chilliness and rigors are very prominent symptoms: "cold hands and feet," "cold down the back," "cold in the whole body," "shivers with cold," "shudders with cold in bed," "cannot get warm all night," "in the evening feverish chilliness over the whole body with a bad cold in the head, but not followed by fever or thirst."

Symptom 440 in Hahnemann is "morning perspiration all over."

This gives a rough outline of the effect of Gold on the healthy human economy as elaborated by Hahnemann and ten other medical men working with him and under his direction. For a full list of its symptoms see Allen's "Encyclopædia." This pathogenesis of Gold is unique, and the outcome of honest conviction, hard work, scientific experiment, accurate powers of observation, unusual love of science and of humanity, and betokens almost heroic self-abnegation.

As far as my reading carries me, a better or more reliable provers' committee never existed for working out the pathogenesis of any drug whatsoever. Complete it is not, neither is it, or could it then be, perfect. We miss the use of the ophthalmoscope to interpret the eye symptoms ; of the stethoscope for the investigation of the hearts and lungs of the provers, both before, during, and after the provings ; the renal secretions were not examined, and the temperature was not taken. Future Regii Professors of Experimental Drug Pathology will fill in the Hahnemannic Cadre, and thus bring it abreast of modern requirements. But even as it is, how immeasurably superior is it to the cat-dog-and-rabbit crudities of the dominant sect in medicine, whose one aim would seem to be to paralyse and kill countless lower animals to see how much a given drug can do and how soon it can do it. These points have a certain value as giving us a knowledge of the last links in the chains, but what we require for clinical purposes is an accurate knowledge of all that drugs can do on the *hither side* of that stage of absolutely lethal organic change from which no recovery is conceivable. These able and honest men are working hard for the science of the deadhouse, but not for that at the bedside. On them the light of the Hahnemannic Law has not yet dawned, and they are still where Haller was.

A somewhat fuller symptomatology of *Aurum Metallicum* than that of Hahnemann (and which includes Hahnemann's) may be read in Allen's "Encyclopædia of Pure Materia Medica," art. *Aurum ;* but nothing was ever done before, and nothing has been done since, on this part of the subject at all comparable to this lasting contribution of Hahnemann and of his ten able coadjutors which I have just endeavoured to portray.

The clinical applications of these pathogenetic facts are to be sought in the homœopathic literature of the past fifty years, and in the numerous examples of *involuntary* Homœopathy in general medical literature.

The Pathogenetic Records of the various *preparations* of Gold, on the other hand, do not commence with Hahnemann, and are only just touched upon by him—viz., he only gives eighteen symptoms of *Aurum Muriaticum*, and three of *Aurum fulminans*. His own idea would seem to be that the pure metal is to be preferred on account of its noble simplicity and superior merits. At first he used the muriate because of its solubility, being influenced by the current literature of the time on the subject, and by those authors who affirm that metallic Gold is totally useless as a medicine because of its insolubility; but then finding that a whole series of Arabian physicians had successively used *finely-powdered Gold*, beginning as far back as the eighth century, and since when *Geber* (de Alchimia traditio, 1698) praised powdered Gold as a "Materia laetificans et in juventute corpus conservans," and probably being acquainted with M.

Chrestien's works, he set about powdering some for himself, and then proved it on the healthy as we have seen. Hereafter he tells us he only made use of the pure powdered metal, therein following the example of the Arabian physicians. Legrand arrives at the same conclusion—viz., that the powdered metal is the best form of administration.

But the salts of Gold are Gold and something else, still their chief effects justify us in considering them, for practical purposes, as Gold; moreover, they seem to give us a deeper insight into the action of the metal on the economy, though possibly only because they have been experimented with to the neglect or exclusion of the triturated metal.

Chrestien's earlier work was with pulverised Gold, but unfortunately I do not possess his earlier publications, and Chrestien's later work—viz., Niel's

"*Recherches,*" etc., 1821, I certainly possess, but being unbound, I fear the greater part of it has served the useful purpose of fire-lighting, as I lately found only a small portion of it cast aside in a corner. But M. Legrand's work will supply its place, as it embodies it in its more important details. It bears date 1828. Hahnemann's first account of the effects of Gold bears date 1825. I cannot quite agree with those who affirm that Hahnemann probably knew nothing of the publications of M. Chrestien on the subject of Gold; and I hardly think it quite sure that he was unacquainted with Legrand's work, though he does not notice it in his *Chron. Krankheiten* in 1835.

For we must remember that Hahnemann may have been well acquainted with Chrestien's work, or at least with the fact of its existence; indeed, it is very possible that Hahnemann occupied himself with the study of Gold partly in consequence of such knowledge. For we read a very good review of the subject in Hufeland's Journal of 1817, i. 117, where Triller's joke about the tincture of Gold of the old alchemists—viz., that it was not *Aurum potabile*, but *Aurum putabile*, is quoted.* Then Chrestien's work is mentioned, and the fact that he used the muriate. Then it is mentioned that in Sweden Berzelius prepared a salt of Gold, and of it Schulzenheim, Gahn, Pontin, and Gadelius made successful use in a case of syphilis. Also that Odhelius had published *seven cases* of inveterate syphilis successfully treated with inunctions of the same remedy, stress being laid on the fact that cases in which mercury had been used in vain

* So, also, Erastus affirms, "*Aurum non aurum.*"

yielded most readily to the action of Gold. Then a successful case of cancer treated by Westring with Gold is mentioned; but other remedies were here used with it, especially *Calendula.*

We may fairly assume that Hahnemann read Hufeland's Journal of 1817 at the time, and as his own experiments are not published till 1825, we can hardly claim any originality for him, and, indeed, he sets up no such claim at all himself. His great glory is that he proved the drug on the healthy, and thus gave it fixity and a scientific basis.

About this time (1812-1820) Gold was used in London and New York with considerable success in syphilis and in dropsy.

To return to Legrand's account of the Medicinal Properties of Gold and of its mode of action on the economy, he says in substance that Gold is an *excitant;*

seeming to act principally upon the *arterial, venous,* and *lymphatic* system. This excitation is always mild at first when the dose is small. A weakened stomach is strengthened, the appetite is at times incredibly increased, and the digestive functions become regulated. The patients feel an *indescribable sense of well-being, they feel themselves lighter* (as they express it), so that we may say that Gold possesses *hilariant properties.* The *intellectual faculties* are *more active.* It has been known to *produce frequent erotic salacity going on to painful priapism.* M. Legrand, however, states that he has not used it as an aphrodisiac, but it has been used as such with success.

By its action on the circulatory system it becomes a powerful emmenagogue. M. Souchier treated more than thirty cases of amenorrhœa with the the Perchloride of Gold, and these same cases had resisted the use of tonics and of many other emmenagogues. (Gold was of old used in sterility and female irregularities.)

If Gold is rubbed into the gums when the stomach is *à jeûn* there ensue *pains in the stomach.* The preparations of Gold also cause *constipation,* but not obstinate; pushed a little further diarrhœa ensues.

The excitement of the arterial system produced by Gold is worthy of special attention, for herein lies its similarity to the *conamen naturae* at the onset of eruptive and other diseases. M. Niel says: "This augmentation of tonicity has for object and result the expulsion of whatever the venous blood may have poured into the circulating fluid and into the lymph."

Gold leads sooner or later to evacuations of secretions that are *preceded* by a *slight febrile state:* the *temperature is raised*, the *pulse is more frequent*, and then follows *profuse* and *long-lasting perspirations* or a *great flow of urine*, or *inodorous salivation* or *diarrhœa*. The *perspirations* have been known *so severe* that the *mattress was wet through;* these perspirations have at times an *alkaline odour*, at times they are *very fetid*. The great *perspirations* are *followed by a gentle moisture* of the skin that at times *lasts nearly a month*. The *urine* is usually *thick, cloudy, and very fetid*.

MM. Niel and Legrand think that this action of Gold causes the elimination of the morbid principle; this elimination being the result of the exciting properties of the metal that *produce a reaction from the centre to the periphery of the body* or *to some point of its extent*.

We know that Hahnemann places Aurum among the antipsorics.

As Barthez says, "*Les mouvements critiques se concentrent tous vers l'organe qui en est le terme.*" Thus, continues M. Legrand, "the existing ulcers and chancres *secrete* an *abundance of laudable pus*, buboes become *vast hearths of suppuration, suppressed urethral discharges* are *re-established* and *existing ones increased; other morbid secretions are at once re-established, eruptions of pimples, crops of pustules all over the body;* so that the preparations of *Gold bring back those symptoms* whose *suppression had caused such serious mischief.* Beyond doubt it is good in syphilis as in so many other maladies to favour the development of external symptoms."

This is a truly Hahnemannic idea. Many thoughtful men have enunciated the same sentiment through all the history of medicine. It is just this idea that lies at the root of Hahnemann's tripartite pathology, especially of psora.

The critical diaphoresis and diuresis produced by Aurum led Dr. Delafield, in New York, in the second decade of this century, to administer it in dropsy, which he did with success, but this had been done long before, as we have seen. The same critical diuresis was observed at the Paris Hôpital des Vénériens.

Dr. Souchier observed the same thing; so also Gozzi (Sopra l'uso, etc.). But I am much inclined to think that the *Sodium* has also something to do with the diuresis and diaphoresis.*

According to Gozzi the perspirations are decidedly *worse at night;* moreover, an excessive dose of Gold renders it a *debilitant* and *depressant;* thus Gozzi has observed *suppression of urine and of perspiration,* exacerbation of the disease,

* Hence the *Aurum muriaticum natronatum* occurs to my mind when *excessive perspirations* are a prominent part of the auric disease picture.

the patients complain of *malaise*, and of *unusual heat*. Gozzi also asserts that *dry warm weather* favours the action of Gold, and, on the contrary, its use is apt to cause inconvenience in *cold* weather, especially cold and *wet*, which, in a homœopathic sense, is equivalent to saying that the symptoms calling for Gold are *ameliorated* by *warm dry* weather, and *made worse* by *cold* and *damp*. In this it is like syphilis itself, and also like the plague (bubo plague).

Reading this, therefore, in connection with its other symptoms, I should class Aurum in *Grauvogl's Hydrogenoid Group.*

Irritable, sanguine, and bilious persons are more obnoxòus to the effects of Gold than the phlegmatic.

Exercise, even fatigue, aids the action of Gold (Chrestien).

Hahnemann affirms the duration of the action of Aurum, when given in not very small doses, to be at least twenty-one days. On this point M. Legrand expresses himself thus: "The preparations of Gold act sometimes for a very long time after they have ceased to be given; besides, the phenomena then produced are analogous to those usually observed during its employment." M. Chrestien cites the case of a scrofulous child, to whom Gold had been administered, and who got quite well of many grave manifestations of the scrofulous diathesis, but an enormous goître persisted. All treatment was given up, and in the course of a year the goître insensibly disappeared.

M. Niel cites the case of a sailor treated with the muriate for an exostosis of the right cheekbone, but it resisted the action of this salt of Gold at the time, and then gradually disappeared in two months.

Schepers (op. jam cit.) thus summarises the effects of the Salts of Gold:—

1. They excite the vascular and muscular systems and may induce fever (Niel and Chrestien; Hermann, Arzneimittellehre).
2. They augment absorption (Zum Zobel).
3. They increase the urine (Plencicz, Niel et Chrestien, Zum Zobel, Vering, Bluff, Bartels, Bourquenod, Delafield "On the Use and Efficacy of the Muriate of Gold, 1817").
4. They augment perspiration (Niel et Chrestien, Zum Zobel).
5. They excite the secretion of saliva (Niel et Chrestien, Zum Zobel, Wendt, Bourquenod).
6. Ingested into the stomach they stimulate its forces and produce a sensation of heat in the stomachic

region, accompanied with increased appetite; if a larger dose be given, they produce pains in the stomach and intestines; they cause nausea and vomiting and even produce erosion of the membranes of the stomach.

7. They move the bowels (Wendt, Vering, Bourquenod, Fr. Hoffmann, Plenck).
8. They bring on the menses (Niel, Carron du Villards).
9. They incite the organs of generation (Wendt).
10. Some are of opinion that Gold belongs to that class of metals, such as silver and copper, which exert a powerful influence on the nervous system. Of this opinion is Vogt (Pharmaco-dynamik).

Thus we see only Hahnemann's proving epitomised, and everybody quoted except Hahnemann, and this is in 1838 in the University of Groningen in Holland. *C'est bien tout comme chez nous!*

But Schepers adds one important piece of information thus: "The Cl. *Sebastian* has informed me that after the use of the hydrochlorate of Gold he has not only seen the salivary secretion increased, but also *the mouth and gums affected,* as is often seen after the use of calomel, *viditque dentes mobiles* atque *halitum oris similem ejus, qui post hydrargyri usum frequens est.* Here it may be stated that one of the oldest uses of Gold in medicine was for the cure of *foul breath!* And one of the auralists, in his anxiety to prove that Gold does not hurt the teeth, says that, on the contrary, it made loose teeth firm again!

If this be reliable, the *inodorous* salivation will no longer constitute a *diffe-*

rentia between the effects of Gold and those of mercury.

I have myself observed very slight salivation and great tenderness of the gums and a pustular eruption result from the Tinctura Auri Mur. 3x, in drop doses four times a day for post-gonorrhœal induration of left testis (from abuse of injections of *Cup.-Sul.*), given with only partial success. *Kali Chlor.* 4 trit. cured the mouth in two days, the eruption in eight, and resolved the induration and cured some obstinate sub-prepucial ulcers in a very few more days. Perhaps too much Aurum had been given, and simply ceasing to give it allowed the cure to effect itself.

I think too much stress should not be laid on the inodorous mildness of the auric salivation, as the statement emanates from the auralists, who are always very anxious to show how virulent the effects of mercury are, and how mild and benign, on the contrary, are those of Gold. We must remember that mercury has been much used and Gold comparatively only a little. A French writer of fifty years ago says: "In England they use mercury as much as we use chocolate in France." Von Schroff thus sums up the Physiological Action of Gold (Lehrbuch der Pharmacologie): "The soluble preparations of Gold combine with the albumen of the body, and hence when given in bulk and concentrated, they, on reaching the stomach, corrode and produce Gastro-enteritis. The albuminate of Gold is soluble in the juices of the stomach and abdominal tube, it thence enters the blood and is excreted principally by the kidneys. The preparations of Gold have great similarity in their effects with the preparations of mercury, inasmuch as they both loosen the cohesion of the organic tissue; they both stimulate the absorbent, secretory, and excretory functions of the skin, kidneys, and salivary glands, and when employed for a longer period they initiate a peculiar metamorphosis of plastic life. They differ from the mercurial remedies in this, that they stimulate more the activity of the heart, and of the blood-vessels, but do not fluidify organic tissue so powerfully as does Hg."

Proving of Aurum Foliatum.

To get a really concrete conception of what a given drug can do, there is nothing equal to *trying it on your own body.* As I, in this, practise what I preach, I made the following short proving on myself.

Jan. 27th, 1879. In my usual health and spirits. 12.15 p.m. Take four grains of *Aurum foliatum*, first decimal trituration, dry on the tongue. This sample was most carefully triturated for a long time. My object in making use of the 1x trituration was to see if our *lowest* trituration had any power. 3 p.m. While returning from St. Martin's-le-Grand I felt *intolerable itching in the right groin in its inner third*, and here was realised the old proverb, *Ubi dolor, ibi digitus*, the street and the public notwithstanding. 4 p.m. Having returned, an inspection shows a wheal, now become tender from the violent rubbing that has been carried on every few minutes for the past hour. 5 p.m. The wheal is gone, but the part remains tender.

28th. Sensations in joints and muscles, like one has after unwonted exercise. Feel very strong, with plenty of go in me. Going upstairs I involuntarily take two steps at a time, and run in and out of patients' houses instead of walking.

Clearly this is the *primary* action of the Gold; its *first action* as an *excitant* and as an *exhilarant.* When will the reaction come, and how great will be the recoil?

29th, Evening. Proctostasis these twenty-four hours, which is most unusual with me and clearly drug-effect. Renal secretion much less in quantity; feel well.

30th. Normal. 11.30 a.m. Take four grains of *Aurum foliatum,* 1x trituration, dry on the tongue. Evening. Very wakeful; well up to work; great mental activity; testes a little swelled and hard.

31st. Last night erotic dreams; early in the morning in bed weary pain in right tarsal bones, shooting up towards the knee. Pains in the bones of skull soon passing off. Astringent metallic taste in mouth; tongue slightly coated with brownish fur.

Feb. 4th. In the groove between nose and cheek a cutaneous lump of the size of a split pea; it irritates, gets picked, scabs over and persists. Feel *not* up to the mark; very depressed and low-spirited; nothing seems worth while. After proving Cundurango several years since, a small wart on my chest increased in size, and it has continued to grow ever since and is now about the size of a split horse-bean, with irregular hill-and-dale surface; it is beginning to lap over and to catch things. Since commencing the *Aurum* it seems a little flatter. The last two nights I have dreamed a great deal of death. 2 p.m. Take four grains of *Aurum foliatum*, 1x trituration, dry on the tongue. Evening. Am unusually wakeful; am told that I look pale.

5th. Dreamy towards morning; am repeatedly told that I look pale and worn; have a dazed feeling in the head.

6th. Feel ill; look pale have pain at the lower part of spine; have had bad nights, dreaming of the dead and of corpses. Take four grains of *Aur. fol.* 1x as before. Evening. Feel fagged, but yet not able to sleep. Feel quite out of sorts. For many days great morbid activity of uro-poetic system; sleep does not refresh; dreams of the dead and of dead bodies. Uncomfortable feeling in forehead; pain at the bottom of spine.

7th. Look and feel ill, and although weary, no inclination for either rest or sleep. Having thus taken one grain and six-tenths of metallic Gold I am thoroughly satisfied that it can make *me* ill. My allopathic brethren maintain that the metal Gold is *inert!* Sure *proof* they have never tried it, properly triturated, on their *own* bodies. *Fiat experimentum in corporibus vilibus homœopathicorum,* say they, perhaps. I desist from taking any more of the Aurum, as I feel so out of sorts, and my memory is so sharp that I fear the secondary effect in this direction might be serious.

March 25th. Still have some pain at the bottom of the spine; the last week or two my memory has been very bad indeed, and I am low-spirited. The before-mentioned wart is flatter and certainly much smaller.

April 16th. Memory a little less clouded; still a little pain at the bottom of back occasionally; the wart is nearly gone.

30th. Memory getting good again; the wart seems again slightly on the increase.

Chapter of Accidents from Overdoses of Gold.

Under this head I propose to narrate a few cases that appear in literature, and offering *most valuable pathogenetic facts,* and rightly belonging to the pathogenesis of Gold; but as the involuntary provers (for these *cases* may fairly be considered as *provings*) were more or less diseased, it is not easy to discriminate the wheat from the chaff.

By giving the cases *in extenso* the reader may judge for himself, and a proper discussion may elicit the truth. Impure pathogenetic observations *must* in part supply the place of pure ones, as the chapter of accidents often takes us to a point of organic change that no healthy voluntary prover would be justified in seeking. I will number them.

First Involuntary Proving.

M. Chrestien was consulted by a young man of 22 years of age, of strong constitution, who had been suffering for several weeks from a syphilitic (we should now use the generic term venereal disease, characterised by two chancres on the prepuce, a bubo in the left groin, and gonorrhœa (blennorrhagie).

The muriate of Gold was administered, beginning with the fifteenth of a grain; before the end of the fourth grain all the symptoms had disappeared, but the patient, unknown to his doctor, took it into his head to administer to himself two more grains, in divided doses, the one into eleven and the other into ten parts. Hardly had he finished the last dose of this when there appeared a *very considerable haemorrhoidal swelling*,* *and a large number of excrescences near the anus accompanied by an abundant serous discharge* (ex ano). M. Chrestien con-

* Legrand here adds this foot-note: "Other observations have offered us examples of *haemorrhoidal tumours* that *owed* their *appearance* to the *exciting effects* of the *perchloride*" (*of Gold*).

sidered this merely extreme excitement of the lymphatic system, and could not recognise any syphilitic (venereal) character in these excrescences.* Presently the *mouth was filled with aphthae,* the *tongue became ulcerated in various places,* and *the hair, the eyebrows, and the beard fell out.* Baths, refreshing drinks, bland diet, and above all the lapse of a little time, repaired all this momentary disorder, and patient became, and remained, quite well" (in Legrand).

Second Involuntary Proving.

A patient who had some chancres and buboes was delivered of them by the administration of four grains of the auriferous salt. Two further grains that he took needlessly, *produced excrescences extending from the glans up to above*

* The protrusion of a hernia (Hahn.) and that of the rectum are of a piece.—J. C. B.

the os sacrum. A few glasses of syrup of *orgeat*, lotions of fresh water, and rest caused these accidents to disappear (*ib.*).

Those symptoms that are in italics are most unwillingly regarded by M. Chrestien as effects of Gold, and referred to the disease by M. Legrand, express, I think, the veritable *effects* of *Gold* IN THE DISEASED.

We call to mind that Pliny already reports that Gold cured warts eighteen centuries ago.*

Third Involuntary Proving.

A goldsmith, a little over forty years of age, after having been cured of a chancre on the internal surface of the prepuce, and of a bubo in the fold of the groin, by means of the muriate of Gold and of soda, then took himself other three grains in too strong doses, not-

* See also the writer's proving of Gold.

withstanding the advice of the physician who treated him (M. Bertrand). During the use of the last grain he had *intolerable itching all over the body;* this was *soon followed by an eruption of tubercules* (little lumps), several of which being *soon covered with dartrous scabs;* these accidents were very *soon complicated with a continual humming in the head and beating of the carotid and temporal arteries visible to the eye; the violence of this beating became extremely annoying, and so violent was it that nothing would calm it;* the *disquiet caused* by it, and that put the *sufferer into constant excitement,* almost *rose to delirium.* The little *lumps* much *increased in size* and they became *as hard as horn;* a beginning *gutta serena* was soon added to this ensemble de maux." It is to be remarked that the patient was guilty of indiscretions of diet, notably making frequent use of coffee and alcoholic liquors, during this prolongation of his treatment (Niel in Legrand).

It would seem then that the effects of Gold are made worse by coffee and alcohol.

Fourth Involuntary Proving.

Baron Girardot gave the auriferous salt for months together in the daily dose of a third of a grain without its producing any other ill effect except *Cephalalgia* (ib.).

Fifth Involuntary Proving.

M. Chrestien gave the muriate of Gold during forty days to a patient; then followed a *considerable swelling of the glands of groin,* although the other symptoms had disappeared; the swelling subsided a few days after the remedy was discontinued (ib.).

Sixth (M. Cullerier, Collaborateur du Dictionnaire des Sciences Médicales). This author thus summarises the ill effects of Gold :—

1. Internal heat.
2. Headache.
3. Dryness of the mouth and throat.
4. Oppression.
5. Gastric and intestinal irritation.
6. Constipation or diarrhœa.
7. Acceleration of the circulation.
8. Fever.

Seventh Involuntary Proving.

Lady. — Gonorrhœal discharge and slight swelling of both groins. . . . Patient was taking the second grain when, one morning, after having rubbed in the remedy (into the gums) *she felt a trembling of the lower jaw and was threatened with trismus.*

M. Legrand attributes this nerve

accident to the too irritant quality of the muriate. She had previously had mercurial treatment, which was followed by hæmorrhoids and fistula.

Eighth Involuntary Proving.

(Absolutely analogous to the foregoing, says Legrand).

Lady quite at the end of her treatment with Gold, in very small doses, *her tongue became stiff and prevented the articulation of certain words;* it went off of itself.

Ninth Involuntary Proving.

M. Chrestien cites the case of a young man to whom the muriate of Gold was given, and it set up a state of nervous irritation; this gentleman, very irritable, had just made use of sulphurous waters in bath and as a drink to rid himself of a rheumatic affection. Then making a venereal acquisition he took 2¼ grains of the perchloride of Gold, which developed a serious nervous affection *with disgust of life, insomnia,* and *augmentation of the melancholy to which he was subject* (ib.).

Tenth (Summary of Accidents by Baron Percy in his Report to the Academy of Sciences.

"We must confess that the muriate of Gold does not always act so happily; in a few cases it had no appreciable effect; in some others it *produced salivation, perspirations,* and *other evacuations.* In several it roused a *general nervous sensibility,* it turned indolent glandular and osseous tumours into a *state of exacerbation* and *inflammation* very difficult to calm. In two patients the muriate (although given in moderate doses and by friction) produced *gastritis* or *phlegmasia of the stomach of a very alarming nature.* In two others we saw it produce *violent attacks of fever and of very severe colic.* Once it *covered the body with a kind of herpes,* after the disappearance of which all the antecedent symptoms showed themselves with the same intensity. A voluminous periostitis, thus far free from pain, was *seized with severe lancinating pains* at the tenth dose, which soon brought on carcinomatous degeneration of which the patient died" (ib.).

It may be remarked that this report was conceived and written in a very unfriendly spirit to the auralists, albeit Baron Percy admits Gold to be a powerful remedy.

Eleventh (Gozzi's accidents are these).

"Sometimes it causes *slight inflammation* of *the tongue, of the gums, and of the throat* (arrière-bouche). Also *inflammation of the cheeks in two cases*" (we shall subsequently see that it cures inflammation of the cheeks).

Twelfth, but Voluntary, Proving of M. le Baron Girardot, who, before administering Gold to his patients, made some trials on himself. He took six grains rubbed into the tongue (beginning with the eighth and finishing with the fifth of a grain *pro dosi*), it produced *very considerable diuresis.*

I have thus given the pure experiment on the healthy first, then the impure experiment on the unhealthy; the latter corroborates the former and shows other valuable effects of a noxious kind.

If we now add the experiments on animals we shall be able to follow the effects of Gold still further, even to their fatal issue. Such a picture of drug disease requires *chronic* cases of poisoning in moderate doses to show not only the *length* of the picture, but its *breadth.*

Who will supply them? We want various kinds of animals kept under the use of Gold for several months to see the effects of chronic poisoning on them.

PATHOGENETIC EFFECTS OF AURUM ON ANIMALS.

Orfila (Toxicologie générale, 2nd Ed., T.I. Paris, 1818) says. . . . Several experiments, tried upon dogs, have proved to me that this salt (*Aur. Mur.*) acts with much less strength than corrosive sublimate, when introduced into the stomach; this does not, however, hold good when injected into the veins; its action is then most murderous.

Experiment First.—At eleven in the morning we injected into the jugular vein of a robust dog of large size three-quarters of a grain of the perchloride of Gold, dissolved in a drachm of distilled water; fifteen minutes afterwards *his respiration became difficult, and wheezing* with *suffocation* and *vomiting* of a *white matter*, floating in foam. These symptoms went on increasing at such a rate that at thirty-five minutes after one o'clock the animal was suffering *great uneasiness*, uttering *plaintive cries* and *breathing with the greatest difficulty. Considerable noise* was heard at *every expiration;* he still preserved the power of walking, but remained *lying* and *changing his position frequently.* At half-past four increase of all the symptoms, and an hour later he died.

Post mortem appearances: *lungs of a livid colour*, except a few *rose-coloured spots; texture dense, like liver, filled with blood*, and *non-crepitant;* put into water they remained just below the surface, only the rose-coloured spots would float, and these were slightly crepitant. Mucous membrane of stomach and intestines sound.

Second Experiment.—Half a grain of the perchloride of Gold, dissolved in two drachms and thirty-six minims of distilled water, was injected into the jugular vein of a small dog; the animal felt no inconvenience; two days afterwards he seemed well and had a good appetite. Being of opinion that the poison had not acted, because it was diluted with too great a quantity of the vehicle, we injected into the jugular vein on the other side a grain of the same salt, dissolved in thirty-six minims of distilled water. Immediately after the animal became *giddy*, he *seemed suffocated*, his *inspirations were deep*, *tongue pendant*, *livid*, he *whined*, *became senseless*, and *died* in *four minutes* after the injection.

Autopsy. Opened on the spot: left ventricle of the heart containing black blood, and was still contracting feebly;

the *contractions* were much *more strongly marked in the right auricle and ventricle. Lungs shrivelled in folds, slightly crepitant, discoloured,* and *hardly floated* in water.

Third Experiment.—Two grains of the perchloride of Gold, dissolved in thirty-six minims of water, were injected into the jugular vein of a strong dog, though of small stature; at once his *breathing became difficult,* the *tongue* and *mucous membrane* lining the mouth became *livid;* he *became giddy,* uttered *sharp plaintive cries,* and *died* three minutes after the injection. A minute before he died the crural artery was opened, and the blood which issued was of a deep red colour, and that part which flowed a few seconds before death was nearly black.

Autopsy. On the spot: *heart* of a *violet colour,* containing *blackish blood* in all its cavities; auricles and ventricles *still contracted at the end of three minutes. Volume of lungs considerably diminished,* their *colour inclining to orange,* their texture *contracted, wrinkled, crepitating* but *little,* and containing a small quantity of blood.

These experiments prove incontestably that the muriate of Gold, when injected into the veins, produces death by acting upon the lungs.

Fourth Experiment.—The œsophagus of a little dog was detached, and a hole pierced in it, through which three grains of the perchloride of Gold in a solid form, enveloped in a small cone of paper, was introduced into the stomach, the animal experiencing no pain. The two following days he was *depressed* and *sorrowful,* but walked about very well. He died in the night of the third day.

Post mortem appearances: *mucous membrane of stomach slightly rose-*

coloured, corroded in three places without extending to perforation; muscular and serous membranes intact; the edges of these corrosions were not black, but exhibited the same rose-colour as the rest of the membrane. Texture of the lungs not hardened; it exhibited a few livid patches.

Fifth Experiment.—A small dog was made to swallow ten grains of the perchloride of Gold, dissolved in an ounce of distilled water; he vomited three times in the space of the first six minutes after the injection of the poison; the matter vomited was nearly all liquid, and in no great abundance. At the end of twenty minutes he threw up a great deal of frothy saliva. Two days afterwards his appetite was good. He ran about and tried to make his escape. On the fourth day he began to *refuse food; he grew lean*, and was very *much depressed.*

He *died* in the night of the *seventh day.* (The temperature of the air was at 3° or 4° below zero, and he remained almost constantly out of doors.)

Autopsy. *Mucous membrane of the stomach,* which was of a *clear red colour,* was *ulcerated,* and as if in a *state of suppuration in more than twenty spots.* The lungs appeared to be only slightly affected.

It follows from these experiments that the perchloride of Gold, introduced into the stomach, acts as a *corrosive,* and that the animals sink under the inflammation produced by it in the coats of the digestive tube.

For toxicological purposes these experiments suffice, inasmuch as they show that death may be caused by the perchloride of Gold in the one instance, when injected direct into the veins, by apnœa ;

in the other, when injected in the stomach, from exhaustion arising from a suppurative process consequent on corrosive lesions of the living tissue, or else from inanition consequent on want of proper food. For it is not shown by Orfila that similar corrosions and suppuration cause death when located elsewhere.

For clinical purposes these experiments teach us too little; we require less acute cases not carried quite so far. For the pathology of the dead-house is not the pathology that we meet with at the bedside, any more than the pretty sights we see *en route* to Paris are those that delight us when we get there. But Orfila's experiments on dogs are instructive, and they were quite justifiable, being instituted not wantonly, but for the benefit of mankind.

Practical Uses of Gold in the Treatment of Disease.

Having endeavoured to trace the origin of the use of Gold in medicine, and then sought to give a rough outline of the effects of Gold on the healthy subject, human and animal, and on the unhealthy human subject, we now proceed to consider its clinical uses.

And first. Is Gold a medicine at all? Are not its pretended uses in medicine a mixture of mediæval and modern credulity and wonder-workings? What evidence have we in the archives of practical medicine to show that Gold has ever really cured disease?

This.

There is not wanting evidence of the use of Gold as a remedy, even amongst the ancients; thus Pliny the Elder describes the use of Gold in medicine in these words (Hist. Nat. lib. xxxiij., cap. xxv.): "Aurum plurimis modis pollet in remediis. Vulneratisque et infantibus applicatur, ut minus noceant, quæ inferantur, veneficia. Est et ipsi superlato vis malefica, gallinarum quoque et pecorum fœturis. Remedium est abluere illatum et spargere eos, quibus mederi velis. Torretur et cum salis grumo, pondere triplici misso, et rursum cum duabus salis portionibus, et una lapidis, quem schiston vocant: ita virus tradit rebus una crematis in fictili vase, ipsum purum et incorruptum. Reliquus cinis servatus in fictili et ex aqua illitus, *lichenas in facie sanat.* Lomento eum convenit ablui. *Fistulas etiam sanat* et *quæ vocantur hæmorrhoides.* Quodsi trito spuma abjiciatur, *putria hulcera et tetri odoris emendat.* Ex melle vero decoctum cum melanthio et illitum umbilico, leviter *solvit alvum.*

Verrucas curari eo M. Varro est author."

Pliny died in the year 79; this account must therefore have been written eighteen hundred years ago. It is computed that his Natural History was published about two years before his romantic death.

Bostock and Riley thus translate the foregoing quotation from Pliny: "Gold is efficacious as a remedy in many ways, being applied to wounded persons and to infants, to render any malpractices of sorcery comparatively innocuous that may be directed against them. Gold, however, itself is mischievous in its effects if carried over the head; in the case of chickens and lambs more particularly. The proper remedy in such cases is to wash the Gold, and to sprinkle the water upon the objects which it is wished to preserve. Gold, too, is melted with twice its weight of salt, and three times its weight of misy; after which it is again melted with two parts of salt, and one of the stone called 'schistos.' Employed in this manner, it withdraws the natural acridity from the substances torrefied with it in the crucible, while at the same time it remains pure and incorrupt; the residue forming an ash, which is preserved in an earthen vessel, and is applied with water for *the cure of lichens on the face:* the best method of washing it off is with bean-meal. These ashes have the property also of *curing fistulas*, and the discharges *known as 'haemorrhoides':* with the addition, too, of powdered pumice, they are a cure of *putrid ulcers and sores*, which emit an offensive smell. Gold, boiled in honey with melanthium and applied as a liniment to the navel, *acts as a gentle purgative* upon the bowels. M. Varro assures us *that Gold is a cure for warts.*"

In a foot-note the translators add, "Similar to the notion still prevalent, that the application of pure *Gold will remove styes on the eye-lids.*" The italics are mine.

It is certainly interesting to note that already at this early period Gold was a recognised remedy in disease: lichens in the face, fistulas, hæmorrhoids, putrid ulcers, and foul sores and warts. Are not psora, syphilis, and sycosis here expressed?

Gold *produces* cutaneous eruptions and hæmorrhoids; the eruptions would probably become sores and ulcers if the proving were pushed far enough. It is evident also that the use of Gold as a remedy in disease did not originate with the Arabian physicians; long before them it was a tradition, and they merely handed it on. Pliny's account of it is that of a compiler, not that of an original observer, and hence Gold was a remedy *before* his time.

Hahnemann mentions nearly thirty authors (1698—1730) who praise Gold as a valuable remedy in various diseases, such as* Melancholia, Weak Heart, Foul Breath, Falling out of the Hair, Weak Eyes, Breast Pang, Palpitation of the Heart, Difficulty of Breathing.

Hahnemann himself used it with success in Caries of the Bones of the Nose and Palate, as an antidote to the Ill-Effects of Mercury, in Hypochondriasis, Melancholy, Tedium Vitæ, Suicidal Tendencies, Congestion of Blood to the Head, Weak Sight, Toothache from a Rush of Blood to the Head with Heat therein, Inguinal Hernia, Chronic Indu-

* We have seen that Gold causes melancholy, weakens the heart, renders the breath foul, causes the hair to fall out, weakens the eyes, causes oppression of the chest, makes the heart palpitate, and renders the breathing difficult!

ration of the Testicles, Prolapse and Induration of the Uterus, Angina Pectoris, Nocturnal Bone Pains, and Arthritic deposits.

Chrestien, Niel, Legrand, and some seventy other physicians and surgeons in France in the second and third decades of this century, used it with great success in all forms of venereal diseases and in scrofulosis (see Legrand). All forms of the former were treated by them: Chancres, Balanitis, Urethritis, Adenitis, Hunterian Chancres, many Syphilides, Sarcoceles, Orchitis, Epididymitis, Ozaena, Caries, Ostitis. The mass of evidence in favour of Gold as an antivenereal is really overwhelming, and that in favour of its use in scrofula is not much less so. But their treatment was sometimes mixed, and not infrequently Gold was administered in cases in which other medicines were clearly indicated rather than this, their pet remedy.

Withal these enthusiastic auralists have brought Gold into disrepute as a therapeutic agent by their absurd prejudice against Mercury and exaggerated pretensions with regard to the antivenereal virtues of Aurum. At first there was violent opposition, then a ripple of professional opinion arose, and soon swelled into a wave that was going to sweep away every other antivenereal remedy ; but Nature does not work in that way, and hence the ebb set in, and the auralists drifted out to sea and were lost in the mid-ocean of oblivion.

One of the most able of pharmacologists and most genial of practitioners, Von Schroff, the celebrated Vienna professor (Lehrbuch der Pharmacologie, Wien, 1868), gives the following case in these words (p. 289) : "I remember a case of syphilis in which the strongest mercurial preparations, such as sublimate, had failed to arrest the onward march of destruction of the nasal bones or the deep, spreading, syphilitic ulcers of the skin, but the miserable patient was restored with the help of Gold" (*Aur.-Mur.-Nat.*).

Speaking of its use in dropsy, especially from induration of abdominal organs, he says: "I remember such a case, that I saw in 'Kromholz's Clinic' in Prague, in which Gold acted as a diuretic and a cure resulted."

The period referred to by Schroff would be some fifty years ago. The grand old octogenarian is a bitter, but honest, hater of the "nihilism of Hahnemann," but we see he is nevertheless guilty of *Homœopathia involuntaria;* and he is also a most successful practitioner.

Dr. R. Hughes says of Gold: "It is an admirable medicine for those constitutions broken down by the combined influence of syphilis and mercury which sometimes come before us for treatment. I once gave a poor fellow thus afflicted the first trituration of Gold. He came back to me in a week's time, looking quite another man, and exclaimed, "Surely you have given me the elixir of life!"

Dr. Chapman has narrated a similar case in the seventh volume of the "British Journal of Homœopathy" (p. 396).

I myself have published in the same journal a case of syphilitic exostoses of the bones of the skull speedily cured with this great remedy.

Thus the traditional efficacy of Gold in syphilis and in chronic hydrargyrosis is handed on from one generation to another in both schools.

The point brought out in Dr. Hughes's, Dr. Chapman's, and Von Schroft's cases is precisely that insisted upon by Baron Percy in his official report of the Committee of Inquiry that sat, on the subject of the treatment of venereal diseases with auriferous preparations, in France fifty years ago.

We may, therefore, consider this point as *proven.*

In *scrofulosis,* Laluette, Chrestien, Niel, Legrand, and quite a host of others, praise it. We find enumerated scrofulous ophthalmia, tinea capitis, scrofulous cervical glands, arthrocace scrofulosa. I believe Dr. Dudgeon, no mean authority, commends it in scrofulous ophthalmia.

Chrestien, in his *Quelques faits intéressants rélatifs à l'emploi thérapeutique des préparations aurifères. Montpellier,* 1835—8 (in Schepers), lays special stress upon it as an antiscrofulosum.

In scrofulous and syphilitic affections of the bones of the nose and face, even of the very worst kinds, and in ozæna, it is much lauded, and when we consider this fact we may well pause, for a more dire calamity can hardly befal a human creature than to be thus afflicted. At present I have one such case, in a middle-aged scrofulous gentleman, that is steadily improving under the use of Aurum foliatum.*

In Von Schroff's case, already cited, there was extensive destruction of the nasal bones, and this remedy cured. Hahnemann used it in the same affection.

We may safely affirm that its efficacy in some cases of this really terrible disease is no longer open to any reasonable doubt. Let those who are sceptical on the subject try it.

* *Kali bichromicum* had been previously administered in vain.

The implantation of the syphilitic virus upon a scrofulous constitution is one of the most intractable of all morbid manifestations, and but few medicines will touch it at all. Gold does. This condition I would term *Psoro-Syphilis*, or *Scrofulo-syphilis*, if I may be allowed to coin an expression to serve the purpose of this paper—viz., to elucidate the curative range of this remedy in this unhappy marriage of two vile constitutional taints. Then, the term being allowed, we may speak of

PSORO-SYPHILIS, OR SCROFULO-SYPHILIS.

Gold seems specially suitable to such forms of syphilis in the strumous; we have seen that Hahnemann reckons Gold to the antipsoric remedies. The glands, bones, skin, nose, are alike stricken with scrofula, syphilis, and Gold.

Speaking of the good effects of Gold in the treatment of syphilitic affections, Schepers reports a clinical lecture of Sebastian, who said, "Auri præparatis non opus est in iis recentis luis casibus, in quibus ægri ab omni alio morbo liberi sunt, sed quando morbus ille in hominibus *scrofulosis* obtinet, in quibus syphilis *facile ad nares transit, ad cutem atque ossa*, tum aurum præferendum est hydrargyro, etc."

Most practical men will subscribe to this. About eighteen months since I treated a baby with "snuffles," and anal and intercrural excoriations ; the infant's nose was dinged in, and she had the well-known ancient appearance. I had previously treated both parents for syphilis (affected skin, indurated glands, and alopecia, the mother's eyebrows even were shed). A six weeks' course of Aurum restored the infant to health ;

when I last saw it it was ruddy and fat.

We may, therefore, do well to think early of Aurum when we meet with syphilis in the scrofulous. In the case just narrated there were numerous circumanal condylomata.

That scrofula itself is sometimes the offspring of syphilis is undoubted. Equally sure is it that the scrofulous are very prone to cancer in later life.

Aurum in Cancer.—Chrestien used Gold in scirrhus of the uterus, but, unhappily, with Cicuta. Westring, Hufeland, Gozzi, Wendt, Helm, Werneck, all affirm the efficacy of Gold in this dire malady. Westring, in carcinoma mammæ et uteri; Hufeland, in cancer of the womb; Gozzi, the same; Helm, in that of the tongue; Werneck, the same.

Scepsis says: Mistaken diagnosis, but why? Gold has strong affinities for the organs affected, so it has, at least, specificity of seat.

Aurum in Dropsy.—We have already noted that it was used in olden times in this affection with success, and in New York sixty years ago, and also centuries ago in Germany ; the case of Schroff has also been quoted.

De Haen and Plencicz gave it in post-scarlatinal hydrops ; Wendt, in the same; Groetzner also in several cases : *inter eos unum, qui locum habuit in viro quadragenario strenuo potatore.*

Fielitz also used it successfully in two cases of dropsy.

I do beg no one will so far misunderstand me as to suppose that I intend to defend the thesis that Aurum is to be given whenever there is dropsy, because this is how medicines get discredited ; myself I should give it in *any disease* whose symptoms showed similarity to those of Aurum, and also purely and simply as an antisyphilitic if only a very few symptoms warranted it. An individual with dropsy, and who was broken down with syphilis, or Mercury, or both, would at once strike me as a suitable subject for Gold.

The following is a case of dropsy of the lower extremities, which came under my observation some two years ago. I was fetched, I think it was one Sunday, to see a lady in Cheshire; it was feared she was beyond recovery. I found my patient, a lady of about fifty, in bed; her lower extremities were swollen, painful, they pitted on pressure, and were worse at night, better in the morning. This œdema had been coming on for a week or two, but it had usually quite disappeared by the morning, and thus caused but very little anxiety, but now it had greatly increased even in bed, and very naturally was causing great alarm. Dropsy is almost always a grave symptom, though not always. In this case I think it was. There was a history of many illnesses, and altogether this drug-picture presented itself:—

1. There was dropsy, and patient had

2. Great depression of spirits, amounting to

3. Profound melancholia.

4. Then there was great difficulty of breathing, and

5. Weak pulse and feeble heart.

6. She was psoric, and had a good deal of

7. Discharge from the nose, that at times contained some blood.

I gave her the Muriate of Gold in the third decimal dilution, but I do not remember the exact number of drops or the repetition of the dose, but the dose was not less than one drop (it may have been two or three), and as often as every two or three hours, and given in water.

The case got rapidly well, all the œdema having permanently disappeared in less than a week. Eighteen months after this she informed me she had never since had any return of the dropsy, though her health was anything but good. This was only a recent case, and, though grave, was yet not severe as to the dropsy, but the despondency was almost a substantive malady.

In this case Gold acted as a veritable pick-me-up, and I submit that the remedy was homœopathically indicated, and the cure a homœopathic one; about the dose I will not quibble; with me the best dose is the one that cures.

It may be objected that as the use of Gold in dropsy is almost as old as the hills, it cannot be claimed for Homœopathy. To this I would reply, Gold will only really cure it if homœopathically indicated; that having a proving of the drug from the hands of that wondrous worker Hahnemann, we have means by which we can *differentiate*, and thus we are enabled to prescribe scientifically. Thus here the symptoms of the case were those of Gold, and patient had dropsy. So a cure of this kind is not merely a lucky hit, or a happy guess, but the outcome of true therapeutic science. The fact that it is in accordance with its empirical use and with authority is of value also, as it completes its history. It is scientific, because Gold covered the symptoms, including the dropsy. Beyond this case, my experience of it in dropsy is *nil*, and *nil* because it is the only case of dropsy I have met with of the auric kind. But has Gold ever produced your principal symptom, *dropsy?*

some one asks. No, not that I am aware of, but it *has* suppressed both *urine* and *perspiration.*

I should use it hopefully in ascites from syphilitic liver. There is a remarkable cure of Bright's Disease with Anasarca narrated in the "British Journal of Homœopathy," vol. xvi., p. 500, effected with *Aur.-Mur.* 6.

Aurum in fistulas.—Pliny already speaks of it (qy. in ano ?).

Case of Fistula in ano.—Young man, twenty-one years of age, bilioso-sanguine temperament. For five months fistula in ano, excrescences on scrotum (eight months after primary symptoms). Cured with five grains of the perchloride of Gold; all the symptoms had disappeared with the third grain (Clinique of M. Lallemand, in Legrand, p. 188).

Another.—Young man of bilious temperament, twenty-six years old, of strong constitution; had chancres, fistula in ano for five months. Cured with five grains of the perchloride of Gold. (Digestive functions excited. Hilarity.) (*Ib.*)

In lachrymal and dental fistulas Aurum is a very likely medicine indeed, for a constitutional taint usually underlies them. In that kind of anal fistula, for which *Kali Carb.* has such a deserved reputation, Aurum does not suggest itself to my mind, but *Kali Carb.* 30 is a grand wrinkle.

Aurum in Hæmorrhoids was, it appears, already a tradition in the time of Pliny.* The brunt of the action of Gold after absorption falls first and foremost on the vascular system. Physiologically it produces piles and greatly irritates the rectum.

One thing strikes me—viz., that there

* Hæmorrhoids, in olden times sometimes signified the *Morbus ficarius.*

must be something rotten in practical medicine when the first surgeons of the day gravely teach, and honestly believe, that piles can only be *radically* cured by operation; when the first physicians of the day are at one with the surgeons on this point.

As a matter of fact piles can no more be *radically* cured by surgical operation than can a hole in the roof of a house be cured by catching the infalling rain in a bucket.

I have never met with a case of uncomplicated hæmorrhoids (I would not deny that more experienced men may have) but could be cured by one, or all, of the following measures—viz., diet, rest, *posture*, and medicines internally and topically.

Topical applications are absolutely needful in *very extreme* cases in which the bowel is protruded very much and the atony of the part is so extreme that the very hypostasis becomes a source of danger and a part of the tumour being thus practically outside the organism. But very few appreciate the value of *posture.*

I find many homœopaths even never attempt the medicinal cure of piles. How wrong and unfair is this to the patient, and, moreover, how cruel! Unhappily, too many medical men "finish their education" when they get their sheepskins; others again use practical medicine as a milch cow and spend all their spare time on a hobby.

Aurum in Skin Diseases.—Of its use in syphilides there is abundant proof; the lichens in the face mentioned by Pliny show how early Aurum was used in affections of the skin.

I shall pass over the cure of the numerous syphilides pure and go on to other cutaneous affections.

Case of Squamous Skin Disease (M. Golfin in Chrestien's Mémoire).—A gentleman, thirty-two years of age, of healthy parentage, and of lymphatic temperament. He has a humid squamous eruption on the left arm and hand. A year previously he had had successively gonorrhœa, the itch, and syphilis, which latter was badly treated. Then ophthalmia, eruptions on the skin of an ill-defined character, and finally dartre (tetter). Depurative treatment for three months, but in vain.

Short course of treatment with sulphur ointment and another with one of the acetate of lead. Then a repercussion from sulphurous baths: hereafter violent cough, causing great distress with copious expectoration and with pains in the chest. A large blister on the arm, tepid baths and sudorifics, reproduce the exanthem, and the pulmonary irritation yields somewhat to soothing and anodyne treatment. Then treatment with the perchloride of Gold rubbed into the tongue and pills of the oxide of Gold prepared with potash, and many other remedies supposed to be auxiliary to the treatment with Aurum.

Patient quite recovered, his recovery being preceded by long-lasting perspirations. Is since married and has healthy offspring.

Case of Severe Skin Disease ; Noli me tangere, by M. Souchier. Alexandrine D——, eldest daughter of an inhabitant of Drôme, enjoyed good health until she was eleven years of age (she is now, December, 1826, nineteen). At this period her father and mother, who state that they have always had good health, were surprised to see her two cheeks become the seat of a peculiar eruption that the physicians, whom they consulted for her, called *dartre vive rongeante,* and which soon made destructive progress at the end of the nose and around its base, notwithstanding the most appropriate and energetic treatment that could be devised for her at Lyons, to which place they had taken her and placed her under the care of the best physicians. Nevertheless the menses set in between thirteen and fourteen ; but this brought no amelioration in her condition, as had been expected. At the age of fifteen all the soft parts of the nose had been eaten away, both cheeks were excavated by the ulcerous inflammation, to the extent of two inches in diameter ; she was very thin, glands of neck much enlarged, so also the submaxillary glands, and those in all the bends of the joints. To this horrible state was soon added all the early symptoms of a tuberculous affection of the chest. Alexandrine continued in this wretched condition till the month of May, 1824, without getting either better or worse. At this period the ulcers of the nose and of the cheeks became covered with pretty large excrescences; those situated on the cartilages of the nose, being transverse, closed up the orifices of the nasal fossæ, and the nasal fossæ were horribly enlarged by the destruction of the wings of the nose. Such rapid progress was all the more inconceivable, as nothing was neglected to thwart and counteract it. Portal's syrup, all kinds of tonics, the most vaunted depuratives, had, as it were, been showered upon her; the most bland diet, and at the same time analeptic, with a view to the state of marasm into which she had sunk, was also adopted. Presently she ceased menstruating and then her parents lost all hope. In November, 1824, a fungous tubercle came in the region of the right eyelid; its progress was very rapid; all the other symptoms of this horrible disease were getting daily worse, when, on the 21st November, 1824, M. Souchier was consulted, who at once declared the affection to be venereal. The coppery look of the wounds and surrounding parts was the point on which he based his diagnosis, and directed him in the choice of his remedial treatment.

Four grains of the perchloride of Gold and of Sodium, divided into thirty, twenty-nine, twenty-eight, and twenty-six fractions, were administered to her successively by being rubbed into the tongue night and morning. After the administration of the fourth grain a change for the better was observed in the state of Alexandrine: her cheeks and all the ulcerated parts of the face, which were dabbed with an ointment of

Gold (five grains of powdered Gold to the ounce of lard, and altogether fifteen grains were thus used), were two-thirds healed. The excrescences, that at first had become paler, grew less, and entirely disappeared at the beginning of the sixth grain, divided into twenty fractions; the fifth had been divided into twenty-four. The fungous growth of the middle part of the right eyelid had also disappeared at this period. At the end of the seventh grain, divided into sixteen fractions, the cicatrisation of the ulcers was complete and her menses reappeared. The stubborn cough, to which the young patient had been subject from her fourteenth year, and which had sensibly diminished from the fourth grain, ceased entirely at the end of the ninth and last grain of the muriate. She got quite strong, and her physiognomy had, very nearly, resumed its former appearance. The end of the nose, although it had been eaten away down to the cartilages, was covered with a very even scar. The cheeks had again taken on almost their natural rotundity, but they have the peculiar appearance of cicatrised parts, and this face, formerly so horrible, is now not even absolutely ugly. It is now December, 1828, three years since this cure was completed, and it still holds good. The girl, whom I see pretty often, *no longer gets the severe colds she was formerly subject to** in the winter months: she had also frequently spit blood.

M. Souchier had at times to cauterise the ulcerated parts when they became granular. When he began the treatment he inserted a seton into the neck.

A more interesting or more terrible case of skin disease can hardly be

* Gold produces a liability to take cold.

imagined, and greater evidence of the efficacy of Gold in the scrofulous it is needless to seek. Therefore I shall tarry no longer under this head. I may, however, just mention that M. Legrand's work contains other such, as well as cases of pustular eruptions, elephantiasis, psora, syphilis, sycosis, and hybrids of the three, and all conducted to a successful issue by the use of this great polychrest. No wonder Hahnemann should exclaim: Gold possesses great healing properties, the place of which no other remedy can supply. "*Das Gold hat grosse, unersetzlich Arznei Kräfte.*"

GOLD IN DISEASES OF THE HEART AND GREAT BLOOD VESSELS.

From the physiological action of aurum it is clear that it must be an important weapon in these diseases, since what hurts may heal.

Angina Pectoris.—The use of various preparations of Gold as a *heart* remedy* dates far back, as we have abundantly shown. That this traditional use was no mere fancy the pathogenesis of the drug renders clear, and it is confirmed by subsequent observation. Hahnemann used it in this serious malady. Dr. Kafka, some years since, published, in the *Allgemeine Hom. Zeitung*, a most interesting case of the successful use of Gold in *angina pectoris*. With me it is, next to *Arnica* (a grand cardiac !), the most frequently prescribed, and it has rendered me most important services. It is here truly *unersetzlich*, as Hahne-

* Hearing of the projected publication of this book, a cruel critic writes and says he is reminded of the Chaucerian—

" For Gold in physic is a cordial old,
Therefore the doctor specially loved Gold."

mann has it. I have seen cases of severe heart mischief, in which Dr. Drysdale, of Liverpool, had prescribed Aurum with marked benefit. I am not sure I did not first learn its use from conversations with this eminent *savant.*

But angina pectoris can but rarely be cured with one remedy; there is often a constitutional taint lying behind and beyond the cardiac symptoms. A case in point just occurs to me. A young married lady used to be seized in the street with indescribable anguish, great oppression of the chest, and fear of death, and violent palpitation. I do *not* affirm that this was a case of true breast-pang with degenerative change. I tried various remedies, hit off from memory, but did no great good. Then I went to work *à la* Hahnemann (of course, I ought to have done so at first; you need not tell me that), and ascertained the *previous history* of my patient. She had had, as a young girl, *an eruption in the bend of her left arm, with rhagades* (Manganese). A truly eminent dermatologist was consulted, because the young lady was going to make her social *débût*, and, of course, required to appear with bare arms. But there was that horrid eruption in the bend of the left arm, and so the *débût* had to be postponed. An ointment was applied; the eruption was—well, sent to the rightabout. She made a brilliant *débût*, soon got married, and began to have a family (once a dead fœtus). She was never well—and her children? Scrofulous. I gave her *Sulphur* 30, and before the twenty-four one-drop powders were used there the identical old eruption was again in the fold of the arm. "Just as it was when I went to Dr. ——;" and patient was at once free from all other symptoms. Patient was so satisfied that there was a causal *nexus* between the exanthem in the arm and her distressing trouble, that she refused absolutely any further treatment for fear it might be *cured* (*!*) again. "I do not mind the arm ; I can wear long sleeves now."

But this has carried me away from the use of Gold as a heart medicine.

Gold in Rheumatic Endocarditis.

In the third part of the second volume of Frank's *Magazin für Physiologische und Klinische Arzneimittellehre und Toxicologie*, Leipzic, 1849, p. 642, we read :—

"*Endocarditis rheumatica.*

"A stout young man who had already had several severe rheumatic attacks, was down with violent rheumatic fever accompanied by painful swelling of the joints. On the second day the rheumatism left the joints and attacked the heart, causing *violent irregular palpitation, with great oppression of the heart.* Five venesections, with the usual antiphlogistic arrangements, got rid of the immediate danger to life; but the subsequent treatment did not relieve patient of his *cardiac anguish,* and hydrocyanic acid would not afford even transitory relief of this anguish (*Beaengstigungen*)."

Then this prescription: *Aur.-Mur. gr. j. Solv. in Aq. Meliss.* ℥j. *Add Syrup. Chamom.* ʒij. *D. S.* Every two hours a teaspoonful. Already the first night (after a few doses) was calm—the first good night since the commencement of the illness. The next day there were only slight indications of oppression and irregular heart-beat. Patient went on several days continually improving, when there appeared a painful swelling of the right hand. The patient felt such benefit from it that he became quite sad when his physician, Dr. Spiritus, discontinued it in order to give other remedies to complete the cure. The symptoms I have italicised show that Gold was homœopathically indicated, though it may be questioned whether Dr. Spiritus knew it.

I call to mind a very similar case of metastasis from the feet to the heart, in a lad who had rheumatic fever, brought on by the nurse putting his feet into hot water. Said nurse exultingly informed me at the morning visit that *she* had cured the feet! The next night there was frightful oppression of the heart, somewhat relieved by Aconite, but it persisted off and on for days, and the poor lad's heart is damaged to this day.

I confess in all humility that I think

Gold was *the* medicine because homœopathic to the state, but unhappily I did not know it then.

Would that we homœopaths kept closer to our study of the Materia Medica Pura, and spent less of our valuable time and talents in internecine squabbles about the precious dose and the eternal name of the school.

I think enough has been said to show that Gold has an important place in the treatment of heart affections of the gravest kinds. But considering the great importance of it in this connection, I will just add very short notes of two other heart cases treated with Gold. They may both be read in Frank's *Magazin*, vol. i., pp. 25, 26. The first of these is that of a lady who, after severe bleeding from the womb, consequent on the expulsion of a molar mass, had *violent palpitation*, *anxiety*, and *congestion of blood to the head.* Usual remedies did no good. Then *Aur. praecipitat* (per fer. sul.) in doses of one-sixth of a grain brought relief after a very few doses, accompanied by this remarkable phenomenon: "*From evening till midnight violent itching beginning in the soles of the feet and then extending to the whole of the body.*" The use of the Gold was continued, and the same phenomenon recurred for several days, diminishing in intensity. After the use of two grains of the Gold the heart symptoms were quite cured.

We have already noted that Gold is an antipsoric with Hahnemann, and in connection with this case the question suggests itself to my mind whether this fore-midnightly itching was a pure pathogenetic symptom or a psoric crisis? *Itching* is a very prominent symptom of Aurum we know.

Now this one more case and then I have done with the cardiac virtues of Aurum. Four weeks after a normal confinement a lady greatly exerted herself and brought on exhausting bleeding; then a few days afterwards there were *rushes of blood, violent palpitation of the heart, great anxiety,* and *faintings.* Digitalis and acids brought no change; then half a grain of Gold was given twice daily with rapid good result.

Dr. Becker, who is the author of these cases, mentions a third and similar case in which Gold was given with the same satisfactory result.

My obstetric friends, how many such cases do you remember in your practices in which you did *not* remember this cardiac action of Gold? I remember one. Cactus relieved it; Gold would have cured it by virtue of the firm grip it gets of the living tissue of the vascular system, and physiologically producing symptoms similar to these.

For Gold is no mere function disturber, but a producer of organic change, and hence its brilliant effects in organic mischief. The vascular turgescence of Belladonna and that of Aurum are very different affairs.

While this was at the printer's the following interesting and instructive case occurred in my practice, viz. :—

Rheumatic Endocarditis in the course of rheumatic fever. I was fetched one day in February (17th), 1879, by a gentleman in the City to see his wife, a lady of about fifty-five or sixty, who was lying very dangerously ill at the end of the third week of rheumatic fever. This gentleman, who is an old homœopath of thirty years' standing, and whose knowledge of drugs and disease is really remarkable for a layman, had treated patient himself, and with no inconsiderable success considering the severity of the case, but suddenly patient's condition became very alarming on account of the rheumatism having apparently seized upon the heart. I found this condition: Patient was propped up in bed and breathing very hurriedly; the lips bluish; tongue dry and coated; anxious expression of face; puffy under eyes; moist râles all over chest, with cough; pulse rapid, compressible, and intermittent; action of heart floundering; loud endocardial bruits; slight dropsy of feet; no appetite at all, could just suck a grape or sip tea; profuse perspirations; limbs swelled and painful, the joints almost as firmly locked as if anchylosed, cannot move hand or foot for pain and from this swelled inflamed state of the joints; flesh of hands puffy; bones of hands swelled, almost immovable, and tender.

I ordered Aurum foliatum, 2nd trituration, very frequently. Alone and no auxiliaries.

Why did I order Aurum? Because it affects the heart and respiration very much *like* they were affected in this patient, and because it moreover produces profuse perspiration, profound weakness, anorexia, and great anxiety. Then the bones were greatly affected.

Feb. 18. A little easier. Rep.

19th. Better in all respects. Rep.

20th. Considerable improvement in the action of the heart; breathing comfortable; is out of danger. Rep.

22nd. Continued improvement. Rep.

24th. Quite comfortable. Continue the Aurum and take Nat.-Sul. 6 trit. in alternation with it. My reason for alternating was that I thought it imprudent to leave off the Gold, and yet Nat.-Sul. was now indicated.

March 2nd. Is up sitting by fire. Appetite good.

6th. Heart, joints, bones, and hands free from rheumatism; is sitting by fire quite comfortably; appetite good; tongue moist, but slightly furred; feet swell a little towards evening.

This is going to press, and hence I cannot give the sequel;* but this case so well illustrates the action of Gold on the organic tissue of the heart that I here insert it.

When I saw patient first I gave a bad prognosis, and had it not been for the Gold I fear it would have been realised. Auxiliaries did not do it, for I used none; faith in the doctor did not cure her, for patient had never seen me before.

* Delay at the printer's enables me to say that patient's recovery is complete; she is now quite well.

Gold as a Remedy in Old Age.

There is some truth in Geber's praise of Gold as a *materia laetificans et in juventute corpus conservans.* Of course it is not literally true, but it has something in it.

Gold will not make an old organism young, but it will do an old organism good, and, *pro tanto,* it rejuvenates.

Last week I saw a lady of some seventy odd summers. She had *great oppression at the heart, cardiac difficulty of breathing, weak pulse, and great depression of spirits.* Her skin showed large *patches of a brown* hue, and again patches like albugo. She was unable to rise. I gave her the third centesimal trituration of *Aurum foliatum* in four-grain doses every three hours. Yesterday I found she had left her bed for a few hours; her spirits were bright, appetite better, her breathing easy, and the oppression at the heart much relieved. "I am quite cheered, mamma is so much better," said the daughter. Six weeks later: She is downstairs, still weak, but very much improved.

The elective affinity shown by Gold for the blood-vessels might make one think of it in incipient atheroma of the arteries in middle and advanced life. I am much impressed with the *visible beating of the carotids and of the temporal arteries in its provings.* In many heart affections, especially in the aged, one sees this.

Before leaving the question of Gold in the conditions of the aged, I will note that I lately prescribed it in a low trituration for an old gentlemen of eighty-five who had severe *attacks of oppression at the heart at night with palpitation and with great debility.* I sent him twenty-four powders, but before they were finished I received the report that "My father is so much better that he is now only taking one powder a day."

It may seem fanciful to some to talk about remedies for old age, but it is not so in reality, for old age may fairly be treated as a disease, inasmuch as it has peculiar symptoms, the like of which are in the pathogeneses of our drugs.

Gold in the Sphere of the Mind.

The efficacy of Gold in Melancholia is, as we have seen, of very ancient date. *Apropos* of this Hahnemann says: "I have cured several cases of Melancholy, similar to those of Gold, promptly and permanently, and they were those of such who went about with the serious intention of committing suicide." He informs us that he needed for the whole treatment about $\frac{3}{100}$ or $\frac{9}{100}$ of a grain.

Here I call the attention of the exclusively high dilutionists to this statement of Hahnemann's. He promptly and permanently cured cases of disease with a one-per-cent. trituration of Gold. These cases are thus on record, and I claim to be a Hahnemannian when I do the same thing. Can *any* cure be anything better than prompt and permanent? I have satisfied myself that Hahnemann's doctrine of drug dynamization is true and capable of scientific experimental demanstration. I honour the high dilutionist as a true physician, and can but pity the arrogance of a crude materialist who denies ability and scientific attainments to high dilutionists because they are high dilutionists.

On the other hand, I cannot but feel that the high dilutionists are very much to blame in their self-assumed isolation. It savours too much of pharisaism.

Militant Homœopathy wants all her adherents, and has a right to their allegiance. Do not let us delude ourselves. Giving crude drugs does not necessarily exclude homœopathicity of drug to disease, and the mere fact of giving high dilutions never was Homœopathy and never will be.

Hahnemann was an omnidilutionist, and gave low dilutions, although it is quite true that he subsequently gave much higher dilutions the preference.

Thus far I have confined myself to the lower dilutions of Gold. When I meet with cases to which Gold seems to me to be homœopathic, and which the low dilutions fail to cure (and such I have hitherto not met with), I shall mount a rung or two of the nosological ladder.

Drs. Chapman, Bayes, and Sharp, all able men, have also treated suicidal melancholy with Aurum with like curative results, as we read in Hughes.*

As everywhere else Dr. Hughes has a theory here too. He says, "Whether this affection is one primarily seated in the brain is doubtful from the other facts about the action of Aurum. I am myself inclined to think it a hypochondriasis having its seat either in the liver or in the testes."

Now the "other facts" show that Aurum affects the brain much more than it does the liver, and quite as much as it does the testes. Hypochondriasis lodged of old in the liver free of rent; it has been many times ejected, and formally located for some time in the testes; latterly it has been a homeless waif. It is satisfactory to learn that its ancient vested rights of

* Dr. A. C. Pope tells me he has likewise used it with great success in such cases of insanity.

domicile are respected. That comes of our living under the reign of law.

Query.—Does hypochondriasis ever sit in the ovaries? or in the *Ligamenta lata?*

GOLD IN THE TREATMENT OF PINING BOYS.

Not infrequently one is consulted about the non-thriving, pining condition of boys; they are low-spirited, lifeless; their memories are bad; they are not up to the mark, and are lacking altogether in boyish go; the tongue is commonly coated at the back, and the appetite for plain food is bad. They are the despised ones at cricket and football, and at school they are not wanting in taste for books, but still they take no position in their forms. "I do not know what it is, but he does not seem to get on." These boys are not necessarily vicious or given to naughty habits, but they are maudlin and unmanly fellows.

Examine the testes, and you will find them mere pendent shreds; just on the verge of atrophy.

A short course of *Aurum foliatum*, 3rd trituration, four or five grains three times a day, seems to act like magic on them; they brighten up, eat, work, play, and sleep like boys should; and their comrades begin to take some account of them in the playground and cricket-field. They become altogether more manly, and spend less time over their books, and yet take better places in their classes. Now look again at the before-mentioned glands, and you will find them larger, firm, and well suspended.

GOLD IN ITS EFFECTS ON THE UTERUS AND OVARIES, AND AS A REMEDY FOR STERILITY.

To treat of this part of the subject is a very delicate undertaking; hence all I have to say is that it once enjoyed considerable reputation in the treatment of sterility, and that I have noticed cases of this condition in which the use of Aurum and of its salts was followed by conception. It is appropriate for such cases in which due ardour is wanting, or where a specific or other taint has lowered the organic vitality of the parts; it is specially called for when want of children has resulted in great depression of spirits.

GOLD AS ANTIDOTE TO THE ILL EFFECTS OF MERCURY.

The immense power and all-sidedness of mercury when introduced into the living body are more or less known to all civilised mankind. To those who know how to use it *in sufficiently small doses* it is no less powerful and all-sided as a remedy. To the disciple of Hahnemann the greater the poison the greater the remedy. A complete symptomatology of Mercurius would fill a big volume with small print.

All authorities agree that Gold is chemically cousin-german to mercury; a comparison of their pathogeneses reveals the fact that they are no less so physiologically. If the effects of Gold are similar to those of mercury the effect of one should be to antidote that of the other. That being the theory on the subject, here are some facts.

Hahnemann used it successfully in chronic hydrargyria.

A severe case of chronic poisoning with mercury is narrated in the thesis of

Timpe (jam cit.) completely cured with the perchloride of Gold in the Charité of Berlin.

There is also narrated a case of mercurial tremor cured with Gold by M. Massel, of Toulouse (in Legrand).

Swediaur speaks of a physician of reputation who was in the habit of using *Aurum fulminans* in the treatment of mercurial salivation, giving three or four grains every evening.

In Legrand, Chrestien, Niel, are a number of cases of venereal affections combined with chronic mercurial poisoning successfully treated with Gold.

To give such cases in detail is needless, as very much of what is contained in the body of this little work belongs equally here.

Our attention is constantly arrested by the remarkable fact that the worst cases of disease cured with Gold had previously been treated with mercurial preparations.

The point has been constantly referred to in these pages, and the number of observers who assert this puts the question entirely beyond any reasonable doubt. Of course it is *not* meant that a case of acute poisoning with corrosive sublimate is to be treated with massive doses of auric chloride; I make this remark because some of the dapper allopathic knights try to *blague* the unwary by falsely imputing this egregious folly to the Homœopaths.

What I mean is that if a given individual shows chronic symptoms of mercurialism pure and simple, or mercurial symptoms with symptoms of any given disease, the chronic mercurialism may be successfully combated with refracted doses of Gold. The utter childishness of asserting that

Homœopathy consists in treating acute cases of poisoning with homœopathic remedies is only equalled by that other pretty assertion that Homœopathy means to grow giants on infinitesimal portions of a bread crumb. An Australian worthy has lately rediscovered this old mare's nest. And he even accuses a well-known homœopathic author with inconsistency for teaching the same treatment of cases of poisoning as is recognised by the authorities in toxicology.

Such nonsense is believed by the simple and is hence noticed in passing.

Nevertheless, even in acute cases of poisoning, *after the ingested poison has been eliminated, or chemically antidoted, or rendered chemically inert*, the remaining symptoms can truly be successfully ameliorated by homœopathically chosen remedies.

GOLD IN DISEASES OF THE EYE.

To those accustomed to prescribe for disease as if it were of an essential substantive nature, or to those who fancy that a given drug possesses a specific benign nature that will meet and neutralise the specific malignant nature of a disease that it is said to cure, the employment of one drug in so many morbid conditions and of various organs, as indicated in these pages, will appear not a little absurd.

Thus I have endeavoured to show that Gold will cure Scrofula, Psora, Syphilis, Sycosis, Cutaneous affections, Suicidal Melancholia, Mercurialism, Dropsy, Angina Pectoris, Inflammation of the Heart, Vascular Turgescence, Cancer, and Specific Indurations. And shall I add now to this long chapter a laudation of Gold as an Eye Medicine? Is it not enough that it should be accredited as anti-scrofulous, anti-psoric, anti-venereal, anti-syphilitic, anti-sycotic? Is it not enough of therapeutic titular dignity for even Gold, that in addition to its thus being a kind of antiomnia it should be a Skin Medicine, a Heart Medicine, a Kidney Medicine, and a discutient of malignant and specific tumours? Will it really do all this, and do good to bad eyes as well? Yes. And let me explain *how that comes to pass*. It is in this wise. Gold will only cure *some* of the conditions of the various parts of the body I have enumerated; it will only cure a *few kinds* of the diseases I have mentioned. Which conditions? What kinds? Herein lies the kernel of the nut: THOSE TO WHICH GOLD IS HOMŒOPATHIC. Now you will observe that I have most of my clinical material, and a good deal of my pathogenetic material, from general medical literature, from allopathic sources, and yet we see that wherever Gold turns up a therapeutic trump, there the *symptoms* of the cases cured by it are to be found amongst those *symptoms that Gold has produced on the healthy.* Do not take my word for it; I may be mistaken. Look for yourself. Compare, for instance, the symptoms of the heart cases I have given (*from allopathic sources*) with those of the drug, and see how very *alike* they are; that is

Like cures like,

no more and no less, whether people have nous enough to see it or not.

Now this Hahnemannian doctrine of similars has been fermenting the medical world for the past eighty years, and although it has not yet leavened the whole lump, it has leavened some small portion, for which humanity has cause to be grateful, and is so, too, as far as its light goes. Unhappily, this homœopathy is nothing like so good as—health! But it comes next to that delightful boon, which most of us throw away when we have it, and then work hard to get it back again.

In a former part of this little work I cited the symptom produced in Dr. Hermann by Gold. It was this: *the upper half of the field of vision seems covered by a black body*—that is, *hemiopia* or half-sight—*the lower half being visible.* That was fifty years ago and more. Now read this:—

Case of Eye Disease—perhaps *Glaucoma*—reported by Dr. E. M. Pease, and which may be found in Allen and Norton's capital work, "*Ophthalmic*

Therapeutics," whose authors are surgeons to the New York Ophthalmic Hospital.

"Mr. I., æt. 24, lawyer, while reading, was suddenly affected with partial loss of sight. Seeking medical advice, he was told that he was suffering from congestion of the retina, and was put under the use of Mercury. After a few weeks of treatment (being twice salivated) he lost his sight completely, January 14, 1873. Received Aconite 12, first three times, then twice per day. January 30. Could distinguish light from darkness; improved slowly to March 26, complaining of fulness over the eyes and floating specks in vision. He received Apis 2c and Merc. Viv. 30m. March 31. His state was as follows:—Feeling of severe pressure from within outward, and from above downward, in both eyeballs, accompanied by dull, heavy aching deep in both globes. On pressure, the eyeballs were more tense and firm than usual. He saw yellow, crescent-shaped bodies floating obliquely upward in the field of vision ; sees a little better on looking intently and steadily at an object, *though he sees no trace of the upper half of an object.* In the *upper dark section of the field* of vision, occasional showers of bright, starlike bodies ; the lower half looks lighter, and he can distinguish colour, light or dark. By gaslight a number of bright, floating specks and dots are seen. Eyes better by moonlight, and after active muscular exercise. Pupils irregularly dilated; cornea dull, with loss of usual lustre ; anterior chamber contracted ; colour of the optic nerve-entrances of a greenish hue, except round the periphery, which was yellowish white, with a slight trace of pigmentary deposit on lower outer edge of optic disc in left eye; the retinal vessels bent abruptly on their exit from the disc, and closely hugging the floor of the excavation, bent sharply upon the periphery of the papilla; central portion of retinal vessels strongly pulsating; large letters cannot be distinguished, he seeing only something black upon a white ground. Aurum was given in the 200th. After three weeks, patient was much improved, could get about the streets alone, being able to follow the cracks in a board sidewalk; the dark half-vision had disappeared, seeing as well the upper as the lower half of an object. Five weeks from commencing with Aurum, everything looked blue, and objects generally much lighter. May 5. He received Aurum M., but was shortly after lost sight of by removing to the West."

Hemiopia.—A man, æt. 52, accustomed to drink whisky every day, has complained for three months of a gradual decrease of vision. At first it appeared to him as if a fog or smoke lay before his eyes; to this, at a later period, black spots were added, and for the last few weeks he can only see the upper half of objects; their lower half seems to be covered by a black veil. Appetite poor; sleep restless and full of anxious dreams; is sad and would cry all the time. Ophthalmoscopic examination gives no clue. Thinking that it was due to the whisky it was strictly forbidden. Aurum cured in four weeks, notwithstanding the patient did not abstain from his accustomed dram.—*Baumann in A. H. Z.*

Hemiopia, in which nothing to the right side can be seen, has been helped though not cured. But the form of hemiopia to which Aurum is especially adapted is when they can see nothing above the medium line, as the following cases illustrate.

Some years ago, a gentleman who had taken large quantities of Iodide of Potash complained that the vision of the left eye had been failing for a year and a half. He could not see the upper half of a room or any large object, though the lower half was clear. No pains in the eye; objects seem smaller and more distant; has some black spots before vision; is always worse as day progresses, and better in the morning; twitching in the upper lid. On inquiry, it was found that he had had syphilis ten years ago, but had not been recently troubled with any secondary symptoms, except that a large bursa-like swelling on the wrist had persisted a long time. Vision was

1880. Upon ophthalmoscopic examination there was found chorio-retinitis (chronic), with an accumulation of fluid beneath the retina, which settled to the lower portion of the eye and caused a large detachment of the retina. Vitreous hazy from infiltration. Right eye normal; refraction normal. Knowledge of the pathological condition here gave no clue to the remedy, and we were obliged, this time at least, to rely upon the symptomatology (as one should be always ready to do). The remarkable symptom of not seeing anything in the upper half of the field of vision is, of course, the most prominent. In addition to the Aurum symptom, we may find under Digitalis, "as if the upper half of the field of vision were covered by a dark cloud in the evenings on walking." Digitalis, moreover, covers the pathological point, having been found curative in fluid exudations of various kinds. It is also worse in the evening, while Aurum is usually worse in the morning. Still, taking the history of the case into account, and the previous dosing with Iodide of Potash, Aurum 200th was given, under which he steadily improved. The haziness of the vitreous almost entirely disappeared, the inflammation of the retina subsided, and in one year the vision rose to and remained at $\frac{15}{100}$, beyond which it will not go, for the retina was partly disorganised, and cannot be repaired with retinal tissue. Since then, several cases of the same disease have been treated with Aurum with almost unvarying success, though in some cases no improvement followed, and the remedy only served to arrest further progress of the malady. Many of these cases will be found to follow overdosing by Potash or Mercury, and perfect vision can never be expected from the nature of the tissue changes.

One singular case of a man, forty years old, was sent for advice. A large black, sub-choroidal tumour was found behind the lens in the fundus, growing from the inner side. He suffered no pain, but the symptoms of vision were those of Aurum (the whole disease had only lasted about six weeks); vision, $\frac{6}{200}$. After taking Aurum 200th a week, vision rose to $\frac{5}{80}$; and in eight weeks more to $\frac{5}{60}$, since which time he has not been seen. It was probably an exudation tumour, and may have been absorbed.

Thus we see that Gold is also no mean medicine in diseases of the Eye. We also note that the high dilutions act as well as any other. So Hahnemann said fifty years ago.

This finishes my task. I have purposely omitted any account of the chemistry of Gold, as that may be referred to in Roscoe, or any work on chemistry the reader may have at hand. I have also said but little of pharmacy, as that lies without the scope of the work entirely. In my practice I have used the *Aurum Muriaticum Natronatum* a little, the muriate a good deal, but I prefer the pure triturated metal. My favourite dilutions are usually not high, but I am nevertheless by no means sure that the effects of the higher dilutions may not be more truly remedial by being more enduring, especially in chronic cases.

I trust the reader may not be less pleased than myself with the effects of *Gold as a Remedy in Disease.*